Managing Cancer Breakthrough Pain

T0093612

Managing Cancer Breakthrough Pain

Donald R Taylor, MD
Comprehensive Pain Care, PC
Taylor Research, LLC
Marietta, GA

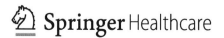

Published by Springer Healthcare Ltd, 236 Gray's Inn Road, London, WC1X 8HB, UK.

www.springerhealthcare.com

© 2013 Springer Healthcare, a part of Springer Science+Business Media.

All rights reserved. No part of this publication may be reproduced, stored in a retrieval system or transmitted in any form or by any means electronic, mechanical, photocopying, recording or otherwise without the prior written permission of the copyright holder.

British Library Cataloguing-in-Publication Data.

A catalogue record for this book is available from the British Library.

ISBN 978-1-908517-76-0

Although every effort has been made to ensure that drug doses and other information are presented accurately in this publication, the ultimate responsibility rests with the prescribing physician. Neither the publisher nor the authors can be held responsible for errors or for any consequences arising from the use of the information contained herein. Any product mentioned in this publication should be used in accordance with the prescribing information prepared by the manufacturers. No claims or endorsements are made for any drug or compound at present under clinical investigation.

Project editor: Tess Salazar
Designer: Joe Harvey
Artworker: Sissan Mollerfors
Production: Marina Maher
Printed in Great Britain by Latimer Trend & Company Ltd.

Contents

Author biography

Donald Taylor, MD, is the Medical Director at Comprehensive Pain Care, PC, and the Principal Investigator for Taylor Research, LLC. He graduated from the Medical College of Georgia in Augusta, GA in 1984. He then completed a residency in Anesthesiology and Critical Care Medicine at Johns Hopkins Hospital in Baltimore, MD. After this, he stayed at Johns Hopkins Hospital for a fellowship in Regional Anesthesia and Pain Management. During his fellowship he established the use of patient-controlled analgesia and epidural analgesia for postoperative pain at Johns Hopkins Hospital. After his fellowship was completed, he remained on the faculty for a year in the division of Regional Anesthesia and Pain Management, providing services in the operating room and in the pain clinic. In 1990, he left Johns Hopkins Hospital and returned to his native Georgia where he entered the private practice of Anesthesiology and Pain Medicine. He has spent the past 22 years practicing pain medicine and conducting Phase II and III clinical trials for pain management medications and devices. His interest in the treatment of cancer-related pain began in his residency when he saw the great relief of suffering that regional anesthetic techniques and skillfully administered medications could bring to patients with cancer. He continues to care for such patients today and has been involved in Phase III clinical trials of several of the newest class of medications, known today as the rapid-onset opioids, developed specifically for the management of cancer breakthrough pain.

Abbreviations

ATC	around-the-clock
BGPF	background pain flare
BTP	breakthrough pain
cBTP	cancer breakthrough pain
FDA	US Food and Drug Administration
FBSF	fentanyl buccal soluble film
FBT	fentanyl buccal tablet
FPNS	fentanyl pectin nasal spray
FSS	fentanyl sublingual spray
FST	fentanyl sublingual tablet
INFS	intranasal fentanyl spray
LAO	long-acting opioids
NRS	numerical rating scale
ORT	Opioid Risk Tool
OTFC	oral transmucosal fentanyl citrate
REMS	Risk Evaluation and Mitigation Strategies
ROO	rapid-onset opioids
SAO	short-acting opioids
SOAPP-R	Screener and Opioid Assessment for Patients with Pain-Revised
TENS	transcutaneous electrical nerve stimulation
TIRF	Transmucosal Immediate Release Fentanyl
WHO	World Health Organization

Glossary

Aberrant drug behavior Any medication-related behaviors that depart from strict adherence to the prescribed therapeutic plan of care.

Abuse The use of an illicit drug or the intentional self-administration of a prescription (or over-the-counter) medication for any nonmedical purpose, such as altering one's state of consciousness (eg, "getting high").

Addiction A primary, chronic disease of brain reward, motivation, memory, and related circuitry. Dysfunction in these circuits leads to characteristic biological, psychological, social, and spiritual manifestations.

Adequate pain control Pain is adequately controlled when it is under "good enough" control to allow the patient to engage in reasonable desired goals. For many patients this will correspond to a pain score on the 0–10 Numerical Rating Scale (NRS) of 0–4.

Around-the-clock (ATC) Refers to a medication given on a time contingent basis over a 24-hour period. The patient may need to be awakened to administer drug.

Background pain Pain that persist for at least 12 hours and usually lasts for 24 hours out of a day (also known as basal pain or persistent pain).

Background pain flare (BGPF) Flare of increased pain that occurs before the background pain is under adequate control. These flares of pain are treated with a rescue dose of regular-release opioid (a short-acting opioid [SAO]). Typically, the rescue medication is an additional dose of the same drug administered ATC for background pain control.

Basal pain *See* "Background pain".

Cancer pain Pain associated with cancer or its treatment. Pain associated with cancer can have multiple causes, such as disease progression, treatment (eg, radiation, chemotherapy, surgery), and concurrent diseases (eg, arthritis, lumbar disc disease).

Cancer breakthrough pain (cBTP) A transient exacerbation of pain that occurs in the setting of generally adequately controlled background pain. cBTP is typically of rapid onset and severe in intensity, and generally self-limiting with an average duration of 30 minutes. cBTP episodes can occur spontaneously or in relation to a specific predictable (eg, walking) or unpredictable (eg, coughing) trigger or incident.

Diversion The intentional removal of a medication from legitimate distribution and dispensing channels. Diversion also involves the sharing or purchasing of prescription medication between family members and friends, or individual theft from family and friends.

Efficacy The ability of a drug to produce the desired therapeutic effect.

End-of-dose failure Occurs when the serum level of an analgesic falls below the therapeutic level before the next timed dose; pain emerges and mimics cBTP.

Equianalgesic A dose of one analgesic that is equivalent in pain-relieving effects to that of another analgesic. This equivalence allows for substitution of one analgesic for another at an equally effective dose.

Intermittent pain Intermittent flares of pain in patients with cancer who do not have background pain. This pain is very similar in characteristics to cBTP, but as there is no background pain, this pain cannot be cBTP or BGPF. Also known as "nonbreakthrough pain".

Long-acting opioid (LAO) Pharmacologically long-acting opioid or an opioid with a modified delivery system designed to provide long-lasting (8–24 hours) relief from a single dose.

Opioid agreement An agreement that defines patient responsibilities when receiving chronic opioid treatment; responsibilities include, for example, the patient's agreement to submit to urine drug testing and random pill counts.

Opioid consent form An informed consent form for a patient who is being prescribed chronic opioids.

Opioid-risk tool (ORT) A written risk-assessment questionnaire (5 questions) designed to assess the risk for aberrant drug behavior prior to prescribing chronic opioid treatment.

Opioid tolerant Patients are considered opioid tolerant if they have been taking at least 60 mg of oral morphine (or an equivalent dose of another opioid) daily for at least 1 week.

Persistent pain *See* "Background pain".

Potency The relationship between the dose of a drug and the therapeutic effect (ie, the drug's strength). A drug is considered potent when a small amount of the drug achieves the intended effect.

Predictable cBTP cBTP that is incident-related and occurs consistently with an activity.

Risk Evaluation and Mitigation Strategy (REMS) A risk management plan that uses risk-minimization strategies beyond approved labeling to manage serious risks associated with a drug. The US Food and Drug Administration (FDA) requires that all physicians, pharmacists, and patients prescribing, dispensing, and using ROOs (respectively) are registered on REMS.

Rescue dose/medication Short-acting opioids (SAO) used to treat BGPFs and used as part of the titration protocol for the ATC analgesic. Typically, the rescue dose is 5–20% of the total ATC dose.

Rapid-onset opioid (ROO) A class of drugs with onset of analgesic action in less than 20 minutes. Currently, all FDA-approved drugs in this class consist of fentanyl and are administered via a variety of transmucosal delivery systems.

Short-acting opioids (SAO) Regular-release opioids that are not pharmacologically long-acting.

Screener and Opioid Assessment for Patients with Pain-Revised (SOAPP-R) A written screening form that predicts the risk of opioid abuse in patients with chronic pain.

Spontaneous cBTP cBTP that occurs without any inciting incident; it is unpredictable.

Transmucosal Immediate Release Fentanyl Risk Evaluation and Mitigation Strategy (TIRF REMS) FDA-mandated educational program for physicians, pharmacists, and patients aimed at mitigating the risks of misuse, abuse, addiction, overdose, and serious complications due to medication errors associated with ROOs.

World Health Organization (WHO) pain ladder Recommendations for cancer pain management by the WHO in a 3-step ladder format:

1. First step for mild pain: nonsteroidal anti-inflammatory drugs or acetaminophen.
2. Second step for moderate pain: add a "weak opioid" (less potent μ-agonist).
3. Third step for severe pain: change opioid to a "strong opioid" (ie, a potent full μ-agonist).

Urine drug testing A test to screen for the presence of administered drugs and the absence of nonprescribed or illegal drugs. Other body fluids can be used as well (eg, saliva or blood).

Preface

Cancer pain management is a broad and vastly rich topic. This book focuses on one narrow, but important, aspect of cancer pain management: cancer breakthrough pain (cBTP). It is assumed that the reader has a passing familiarity with acute and chronic cancer pain and its management, but would like to have a better understanding of cBTP and the new class of drugs – the rapid-onset opioids (ROOs) – developed specifically for the management of cBTP.

The purpose of this book is to provide healthcare professionals with clinically relevant information for understanding and managing cBTP. Early chapters will discuss the history of cBTP treatment and will explain a practical definition of cBTP suitable for caring for the patient with cancer. Subsequent chapters will be devoted to reviewing assessment techniques and widely accepted treatment recommendations for cBTP. Particular emphasis will be placed on current state-of-the-art medications (ie, ROOs) approved for the management of cBTP. The risks associated with ROOs, including abuse, diversion, and addiction, will be explored as well. Lastly, the book will explain the federally mandated Risk Evaluation and Mitigation Strategies (REMS), and how REMS plays a role in attenuating some of the risks associated with ROOs.

The author hopes that this concise book will help fill some of the gaps in knowledge that may exist with regards to cBTP and its treatment.

Chapter 1

Introduction

Experiencing the multidimensional aspects of pain as a patient with cancer

The impact of pain on patients with cancer should not be underestimated. Pain is the most common symptom associated with cancer [1–3]; the reported prevalence of cancer breakthrough pain (cBTP) is as high as 51–89% [4–6]. In patients with solid tumors, up to 75% will have significant chronic pain [7], and almost 70% of patients with terminal cancer experience unrelieved pain [8]. Cancer pain may be neuropathic, nociceptive, or mixed neuropathic–nociceptive. Nociceptive pain syndromes may be visceral or somatic, whereas neuropathic pain syndromes may be central (brain and spinal cord) or related to the peripheral nervous systems. Furthermore, cancer treatments (eg, surgery, chemotherapy, radiation) can be sources of pain. Thus, there are many anatomical substrates for cancer pain [9].

Pain is second only to incurability among the factors people fear most about the diagnosis of cancer [10]. Chronic pain imposes a burden upon many types of patients, but for patients with cancer it is often a metaphor for impending death [11]. In my clinical experience, patients with cancer have told me that when they are not having pain they can forget for a while that they have cancer. This gives special meaning to the management of cancer pain as patients suffer not just from the pain itself but from the message of the pain: they may be at the end-of-life [12].

Chronic cancer pain has been shown to be associated with clinically important depressive symptoms and psychological distress as well [3].

D. R. Taylor., *Managing Cancer Breakthrough Pain*,
DOI: 10.1007/978-1-908517-83-8_1, © Springer Healthcare 2013

Suffering follows from the emotional reaction to the pain and may assail patients with cancer as they struggle to accept their diagnosis. Financial and family stressors may introduce altered social structure that may cause additional suffering [13,14]. In brief, cancer pain can be complicated with physical, psychological, spiritual, and social dimensions [15,16], and management of pain in patients with cancer should be part of a larger strategy of physical, psychological, social, and spiritual end-of-life care [9].

Cancer pain is often poorly managed

Healthcare professionals who care for patients with cancer should be familiar with the management of cancer-related pain since cancer pain is common. Unfortunately, studies suggest that cancer pain is often poorly managed [17–19] and that physician training is deficient when it comes to cancer-pain management [20]. In 2011, a study based in Italy, reporting on 1801 cases, found that 40.3% of patients with cancer presented with cBTP at baseline oncologic- or palliative-care evaluations and that most of these patients were not receiving rescue medications; this study confirmed the prevalence and substantial under-treatment of cBTP [21]. Another study that investigated patients with terminal cancer in a hospice in the UK, reported that 89% of patients who were admitted to the hospice suffered from cBTP and that 75% of these patients were dissatisfied with their pain control [6]. A recent study from an oncology treatment center in the United States showed that 33% of 2026 patients with cancer pain were receiving inadequate analgesic prescribing [22]. In another study from the United States, 42% of 597 patients with cancer pain were not given sufficient analgesic therapy [23]. Under-treatment of cancer pain is a worldwide problem; a review of the literature that included articles from Europe, Asia, and the United States showed that nearly one of two patients experiencing cancer pain was under-treated [17].

Historical perspective

The World Health Organization's pain ladder

There was no universally accepted approach for cancer pain management prior to the World Health Organization (WHO)'s "pain ladder", developed approximately a quarter of a century ago (Figure 1.1) [24–26].

Clinicians often reserved opioids for actively dying patients and, in general, cancer pain was poorly managed [14,27]. Opiophobia, or a fear of opioids, may have played a role in this failure of physicians to adequately control cancer pain [28,29]; opiophobia is an irrational and undocumented fear that appropriate opioid use will lead patients to become addicts [28]. There was great concern about the possibility of causing addiction, even at the end-of-life, and there was also fear that the use of opioids might hasten death. This coupled with the fear of causing addiction often led to the under-treatment of cancer pain [30]. In recognition of the under-treatment of cancer pain, in 1986, the WHO launched a worldwide initiative to improve cancer pain management [31,32].

The WHO also summarized key concepts of cancer pain treatment by describing medications as:
- "by mouth";
- "by the clock" or around-the-clock (ATC);
- "by the ladder";
- "for the individual"; and
- with "attention to detail".

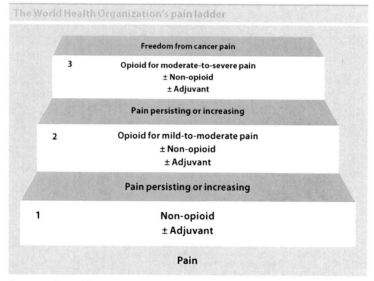

Figure 1.1 The World Health Organization's pain ladder. Three-step analgesic ladder for the management of cancer pain. Adapted from World Health Organization [24].

One of the key concepts put forth in this initiative was the use of opioids "by the clock", or ATC, to treat any patient with cancer who had moderate-to-severe pain, not just for patients who were terminally ill. The ATC approach suggests that analgesics should be administered at fixed intervals of time throughout the day to adequately control background or ATC pain; the time intervals should be such that the analgesic effect from the previous dose does not wear off prior to the administration of the next dose [24]. This "by the clock" or ATC approach to opioid dosing for cancer pain has since been adopted by many medical communities around the world [33]. As discussed later, the ATC opioid also plays a crucial role in determining cBTP and how it should be treated.

The term "by the mouth" simply refers to the fact that the oral route is one of the easiest and most accepted routes for drug delivery; thus, drugs for pain are most often given "by the mouth". However, for a variety reasons other routes may be needed and should be used if the oral route is unacceptable [24].

The "by the ladder" approach refers to the WHO's three-step paradigm (see Figure 1.1) for the management of cancer pain. The first step on the ladder represents treatment recommendations for mild pain (ie, a Numerical Rating Scale [NRS] score of 1–3 on the 0–10 scale [Figure 1.2]), which may be treated by nonsteroidal anti-inflammatory drugs or acetaminophen. The second step on the ladder is for moderate pain (NRS score of 4–6), which may be managed with a "weak opioid", such as codeine and analgesic adjuvants (eg, tricyclic antidepressants, anticonvulsants) that are added to the overall pharmacologic treatment of cancer pain. The third step is for severe pain (NRS score of 7–10), where a "strong opioid", such as morphine, is added to the regimen [14,24,34]. It is beyond the scope of this book to cover the general pharmacologic treatment of cancer pain in detail; however, the reader should be aware that the simple WHO pain ladder approach to cancer pain management is effective in the majority of patients with cancer pain [32].

The terms "for the individual" allude to the fact that each patient with cancer pain is an individual and that treatment needs to be tailored for each and every patient; one drug or one dose does not fit all. The general rule is to titrate medications until an adequate effect is reached.

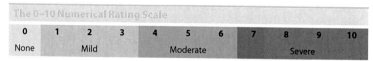

Figure 1.2 The 0–10 Numerical Rating Scale. Adapted from McCaffery et al [34].

Treatment also needs to proceed with "attention to detail". Side effects, such as sedation, nausea, and constipation, need to be monitored and treated aggressively [24].

The around-the-clock opioid

When the WHO initiative was launched, morphine was the most widely available "strong opioid" and initially was used as a liquid or regular-release tablet typically given every 4 hours ATC. The first long-acting opioid (LAO), an extended-release morphine preparation, was approved by the US Food and Drug Administration (FDA) in 1987, and is prescribed on an every 8 to 12 hour basis for the relief of moderate-to-severe pain. The introduction of this long-acting drug reduced the burden on the patient with cancer and their caregivers. The patient did not need to be awakened every 4 hours and the caregiver was not required to administer a pain medication every 4 hours [14,35]. Morphine and extended-release morphine are mentioned here simply because of their historic role in cancer pain management [31]. A detailed discussion of ATC medications used as basal or background analgesics is beyond the scope of this book; however, an understanding of how the background analgesic is dosed (titrated-to-effect) is necessary to understand the historical development of cBTP and its treatment. Today there are many LAOs available as ATC medications for cancer pain; morphine, fentanyl, hydromorphone, oxycodone, oxymorphone, tapentadol, and buprenorphine are all available in extended-release preparations.

The individualization of dosing requires titration of the ATC opioid in order to achieve the optimal effect for each patient. For safety, one such titration scheme is to start the patient on a standard dose of a regular-release opioid (also known as a short-acting opioid [SAO]), such as morphine ATC (to include awakening the patient, if necessary). The patient is also allowed to take a fraction of the ATC dose on an as-needed basis as

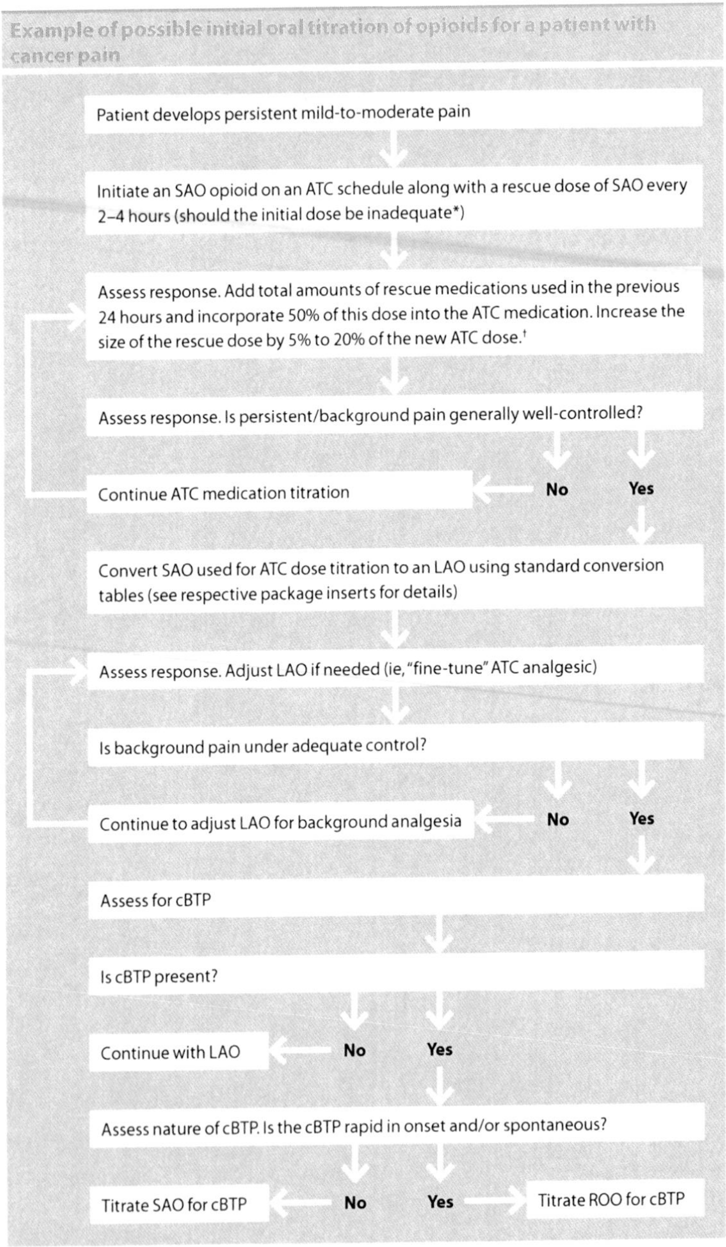

Example of possible initial oral titration of opioids for a patient with cancer pain

Patient develops persistent mild-to-moderate pain

↓

Initiate an SAO opioid on an ATC schedule along with a rescue dose of SAO every 2–4 hours (should the initial dose be inadequate*)

↓

Assess response. Add total amounts of rescue medications used in the previous 24 hours and incorporate 50% of this dose into the ATC medication. Increase the size of the rescue dose by 5% to 20% of the new ATC dose.†

↓

Assess response. Is persistent/background pain generally well-controlled?

↓

Continue ATC medication titration ← **No**   **Yes**

↓

Convert SAO used for ATC dose titration to an LAO using standard conversion tables (see respective package inserts for details)

↓

Assess response. Adjust LAO if needed (ie, "fine-tune" ATC analgesic)

↓

Is background pain under adequate control?

↓

Continue to adjust LAO for background analgesia ← **No**   **Yes**

↓

Assess for cBTP

↓

Is cBTP present?

↓

Continue with LAO ← **No**   **Yes**

↓

Assess nature of cBTP. Is the cBTP rapid in onset and/or spontaneous?

↓

Titrate SAO for cBTP ← **No**   **Yes** → Titrate ROO for cBTP

Figure 1.3 Example of possible initial oral titration of opioids for a patient with cancer pain (caption continued opposite).

a rescue dose [14,35]. The amount of medication utilized for rescue in a 24-hour period is then incorporated into the total daily dose for the next 24 hours and given as part of the ATC medication [14,16]. This process is repeated daily until the pain is controlled by the ATC medication and further rescue doses are not needed or are only rarely needed (Figure 1.3); the total daily dose of the SAO can then be converted to an LAO with the dosing frequency appropriately adjusted [16,35]. At the end of titration (ie, after the ATC medication is converted to an LAO) patients are allowed a rescue dose of a regular-release opioid, such as morphine elixir every 2 hours on an as-needed basis, in case there are still flares of pain [35].

The size of the rescue dose used during and after background analgesic titration is usually 5–20% of the total daily dose and should be available every 2 hours [9,36]. After titration, the rescue medication should be needed infrequently. Typically, titration is considered successful if rescue doses are needed less than 3–4 times per day [35,38]. Indeed, if the patient requires more than 3 rescue doses in a 24-hour period, physicians should consider increasing the ATC medication [38]. The goal of background analgesic titration is complete pain relief; however, this is not always possible and patients may have to accept some persistent pain of generally only mild-to-moderate intensity.

This approach to titration of the ATC pain medication would seem to solve the problem of cancer pain management; nevertheless, as the 24-hour ATC dose is increased, some patients will become sedated or have other side effects [27,35]. One strategy to reduce sedation is to reduce the ATC dose and use rescue doses as needed [39].

Figure 1.3 Example of possible initial oral titration of opioids for a patient with cancer pain (continued). This is a common example of an opioid titration scheme; however, this is not the only possible option. This example should acquaint the reader with the process of opioid titration for managing patients with cancer pain. *For example, a patient prescribed an SAO 15 mg/4 hrs ATC (eg, morphine tablets at 90 mg/day) may have an additional dose (eg, 5 mg/2 hrs), if needed, as a rescue medication; SAO rescue medications are usually 5–20% of total daily dose, which should be held or lowered if sedation or if an adverse event occurs; †rounding may be required to easily utilize commercial preparations. Prescriptions for rescue doses might also be increased to 5–20% of the new total daily dose. These calculations can be repeated daily until pain is under stable control. Once the basal pain is under adequate control, the ATC medication may be converted to an LAO for the comfort and convenience of the patient and caregiver [35]. ATC, around-the-clock; cBTP, cancer breakthrough pain; LAO, long-acting opioid; ROO, rapid-onset opioid; SAO, short-acting opioid. Data from Caraceni et al [9], Portenoy et al [15], Coyle et al [36], and National Cancer Institute [37].

Pain flares and their treatment

After titration of the ATC medication, some patients may have generally well-controlled pain most of the day but may experience episodic flares of moderate-to-severe pain that break through their ATC analgesic control [40,41]. Some of these pain flares may occur spontaneously, rapidly develop to maximal intensity, and be relatively short in duration, generally lasting less than 1 hour [41,42]. In the past, the typical drugs used for rescue medication, such as morphine, did not always work well for treating these pain flares as their time course of action did not match the time course of the pain. These drugs did not always provide relief until after the pain was mostly abated [43]. Figure 1.4 shows the temporal mismatch that can occur between the peak of the cBTP flare and the SAO taken at the onset of the pain flare [34,44].

A preferred medication to treat the flares of pain that break through the background or ATC analgesic would be one that perfectly matches

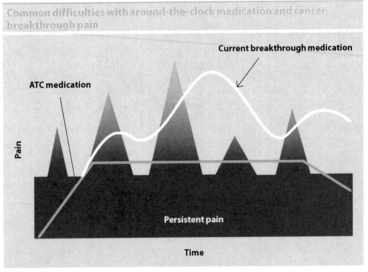

Figure 1.4 Common difficulties with around-the-clock medication and cancer breakthrough pain. The ATC (green line) medication controls the persistent/background pain (red rectangle). The flares of cBTP (orange peaks) break through the ATC medication. The SAO (white line) effect peaks after the flare of cBTP subsides. This mismatch between the temporal profile of the cBTP flare and the cBTP medication can lead to excessive sedation when the peak effect of the opioid is not opposed by pain. ATC, around-the-clock; cBTP, cancer breakthrough pain, SAO, short-acting opioids. Adapted from Bennett et al [44].

the intensity and temporal profile of the pain flares [44]; such a model cBTP medication is illustrated in Figure 1.5 [44]. A medication that exactly fits this model, however, does not yet exist.

Some years ago researchers in cancer pain management began to recognize the need to match the analgesic regimen to the temporal pain profile. Predictable flares of pain, such as from a particular movement, could be treated by administering a rescue medication approximately 30 minutes to 1 hour prior to the painful event. However, it was the unpredictable episodes of pain that were the most problematic, and these episodes turned out to be surprisingly frequent [4]. At the time there were no oral analgesics available that could match the time course of these unpredictable, spontaneous and rapidly escalating, short-duration flares of pain [41], and pre-emptive analgesic approaches were not optimal for their management [44]. It was not until the rapid-onset opioids (ROOs) were developed that the oral management of cBTP became feasible; until this milestone in pain medicine occurred, only intravenous opioids could match the time course of spontaneous cBTP episodes [45].

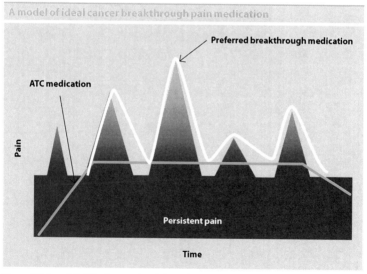

Figure 1.5 A model of ideal cancer breakthrough pain medication. This figure illustrates how the ideal cBTP medication would perfectly match the time course of the cBTP episode. Low-intensity pain flares would respond to one dose; high-intensity pain flares would respond to several doses. ATC, around-the-clock; cBTP, cancer breakthrough pain. Adapted from Bennett et al [44].

The rapid-onset opioids arrive

In an attempt to improve upon the time course of the traditional SAO or rescue medications, the ROOs were developed to better match the time course of a patient's cBTP episode [9,46]. The introduction of oral transmucosal fentanyl citrate (OTFC), the first ROO, gave clinicians the first drug whose time course of action mimicked the time-intensity profile of cBTP (Figure 1.6) [47]. ROOs tend to produce an onset of analgesia in as little as 5–15 minutes. This means that with a ROO, compared to standard SAOs, patients can obtain more timely relief from the sometimes excruciating spikes of spontaneous cBTP. With the introduction of a medication to treat spontaneous cBTP, research into the nature and treatment of cBTP blossomed and in the last few years a number of ROOs have been approved for the management of cBTP.

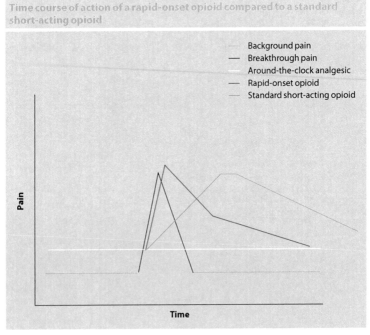

Figure 1.6 Time course of action of a rapid-onset opioid compared to a standard short-acting opioid. For spontaneous rapidly escalating flares of cancer breakthrough pain, the time course of action of the rapid-onset opioid matches the pain profile more accurately than the short-acting opioid.

References

1   Cleeland CS. The impact of pain on the patient with cancer. *Cancer*. 1984;54 (11 Suppl):2635-2641.

2   Schrijvers D. Pain control in cancer: recent findings and trends. *Ann Oncol.* 2007;18(9 Suppl):ix37-ix42.

3   Green CR, Montague L, Hart-Johnson TA. Consistent and breakthrough pain in diverse advanced cancer patients: a longitudinal examination. *J Pain Symptom Manage*. 2009;37:831-847.

4   Portenoy RK, Payne D, Jacobsen P. Breakthrough pain: characteristics and impact in patients with cancer pain. *Pain*. 1999;81:129-134.

5   Caraceni A, Martini C, Zecca E, et al; Working Group of an IASP Task Force on Cancer Pain. Breakthrough pain characteristics and syndromes in patients with cancer pain. An international survey. *Palliat Med*. 2004;18:177-183.

6   Zeppetella G, O'Doherty CA, Collins S. Prevalence and characteristics of breakthrough pain in cancer patients admitted to a hospice. *J Pain Symptom Manage*. 2000;20:87-92.

7   Goudas LC, Bloch R, Gialeli-Goudas M, Lau J Carr DB. The epidemiology of cancer pain. *Cancer Invest*. 2005;23:182-190.

8   Carr D, Goudas L, Lawrence D, et al. Management of cancer symptoms: pain, depression, and fatigue. Agency for Healthcare and Research Quality. New England Medical Center Evidence-based Practice Center. archive.ahrq.gov/downloads/pub/evidence/pdf/cansymp/cansymp.pdf. Published July 2002. Accessed February 1, 2013.

9   Caraceni A, Martin C, Zecca E, Fagnoni E. Cancer pain management and palliative care. In: Grisold W, Soffietti R, eds. *Handbook of Clinical Neurology*. 3rd ed. New York, NY: Elsevier; 2012:391-415.

10 Ahles TA, Blanchard EB, Ruckdeschel JC. The multidimensional nature of cancer-related pain. *Pain*. 1983;17:277-288.

11 Ferrell BR, Dean G. The meaning of cancer pain. *Semin Oncol Nurs*. 1995;11:17-22.

12 Webber K, Davies AN, Cowie MR. Breakthrough pain: a qualitive study involving patients with advanced cancer. *Support Care Cancer*. 2011;19:2041-2046.

13 Cherny NI, Coyle N, Foley KM. Suffering in the advanced cancer patient: a definition and taxonomy. *J Palliat Care*. 1994;10:57-70.

14 Bonica JJ, Ekstrom JL. Systemic Opioids for the management of cancer pain: an updated review. In: Bendetti C, ed. *Advances in Pain Research and Therapy*. Volume 14. New York, NY: Raven Press, Ltd; 1990:425-446.

15 Portenoy RK. Treatment of cancer pain. *Lancet*. 2011;377:2236-2247.

16 McGuire D. The multiple dimensions of cancer pain: a framework for assessment and management. In: McGuire D, Yarbro CH, Ferrell BR. 2nd ed. *Cancer Pain Management*. Boston, MA: Jones and Bartlett Publishers; 1995:1-17.

17 Deandrea S, Montanari M, Moja L, Apolone G. Prevalence of undertreatment in cancer pain. A review of published literature. *Ann Oncol*. 2008;19:1985-1991.

18 Apolone G, Corli O, Caraceni A, et al; Cancer Pain Outcome Research Study Group (CPOR SG) Investigators. Pattern and quality of care of cancer pain management. Results from the Cancer Pain Outcome Research Study Group. *Br J Cancer*. 2009;100:1566-1574.

19 Lossignol DA, Dumitrescu C. Breakthrough pain: progress in management. *Curr Opin Oncol*. 2010;22:302-306.

20 Mortimer JE, Bartlett NL. Assessment of knowledge about cancer pain management by physicians in training. *J Pain Symptom Manage*. 1997;14:21-28.

21 Greco MT, Corli O, Montanari M, Deandrea S, Zagonel V, Apolone G; Writing Protocol Committee; Cancer Pain Outcome Research Study Group (CPOR SG) Investigators. Epidemiology and pattern of care of breakthrough cancer pain in a longitudinal sample of cancer patients: results from the Cancer Pain Outcome Research Study Group. *Clin J Pain*. 2011;27:9-18.

22 Fisch MJ, Lee JW, Weiss M, et al. Prospective, observational study of pain and analgesic prescribing in medical oncology outpatients with breast, colorectal, lung, or prostate cancer. *J Clin Oncol*. 2012;30:1980-1988.

23 Cleeland CS, Gonin R, Hatfield AK, et al. Pain and its treatment in outpatients with metastatic cancer. *N Engl J Med*. 1994;330:592-596.

24 World Health Organization. Cancer pain relief second edition with a guide to opioid availability. whqlibdoc.who.int/publications/9241544821.pdf. Published 1996. Accessed February 1, 2013.

25 Stjernswärd J. WHO cancer pain relief programme. *Cancer Surv*. 1988;7:195-208.

26 Seymour J, Clark D, Winslow, M. Pain and palliative care: the emergence of new specialties. *J Pain Symptom Manage*. 2005;29:2-13.

27 Ventafridda V, Tamburini M, Caraceni A, De Conno F, Naldi F. A validation study of the WHO method for cancer pain relief. *Cancer*. 1987;59:850-856.

28 Morgan JP. American opiophobia: customary underutilization of opioid analgesics. *Adv Alcohol Subst Abuse*. 1985;5:163-173.

29 Rhodin A. The rise of opiophobia: is history a barrier to prescribing? *J Pain Palliat Care Pharmacother*. 2006;20:31-32.

30 Fohr SA. The double effect of pain medication: separating myth from reality. *J Palliat Med*. 1998;1:315-328.

31 Meldrum M. The ladder and the clock: cancer pain and public policy at the end of the twentieth century. *J Pain Symptom Manage*. 2005;29:41-54.

32 Zech DF, Grond S, Lynch J, Hertel D, Lehmann KA. Validation of World Health Organization Guidelines for cancer pain relief: a 10-year prospective study. *Pain*. 1995;63:65-76.

33 World Health Organization. Pain & Palliative Care Communications Program. 2005;18.

34 McCaffery M, Beebe A. *Pain: Clinical Manual for Nursing Practice*. Baltimore, MD: V.V. Mosby Company; 1993.

35 Levy MH. Oral controlled release morphine: guidelines for clinical use. In: Bendetti C, ed. *Advances in Pain Research and Therapy*. New York, NY: Raven Press, Ltd; 1990:285-295.

36 Coyle N, Cherny N, Portenoy RK. Pharmacologic management of cancer pain. In: McGuire DB, Yarbro CH, Ferrel BR. *Cancer Pain Management*. 2nd ed. Boston, MA: Jones and Barlett Publishers; 1995:89-130.

37 National Cancer Institute. Pain (PDQ®) Health Professional Version. www.cancer.gov/cancertopics/pdq/supportivecare/pain/HealthProfessional/page1. Accessed February 1, 2013.

38 Hill CS. Oral opioid analgesics. In Patt RB, ed. *Cancer Pain*. Philadelphia, PA: J.B. Lippincott Company; 1993:129-142.

39 Portenoy RK. *Contemporary Diagnosis and Management of Pain in Oncologic and AIDS Patients*. Newton, PA: Handbooks in Health Care Company; 1997:119-120.

40 Portenoy RK, Hagen NA. Breakthrough pain: definition, prevalence and characteristics. *Pain*. 1990;41:273-281.

41 Portenoy RK, Hagen NA. Breakthrough pain: definition and management. *Oncology (Williston Park)*. 1989;3(8 Suppl):25-29.

42 Davies A, Zeppetella G, Andersen S, et al. Multi-centre European study of breakthrough cancer pain: pain characteristics and patient perceptions of current and potential management strategies. *Eur J Pain*. 2011;15:756-763.

43 Zeppetella G. Opioids for cancer breakthrough pain: a pilot study reporting patient assessment of time to meaningful pain relief. *J Pain Symptom Manage*. 2008;35:563-567.

44 Bennett D, Burton AW, Fishman S, et al. Consensus panel recommendations for the assessment and management of breakthrough pain: Part 2 Management. *P T*. 2005;30:354-361.

45 Fine PG. Advances in cancer pain management. In: Lake CL, Rice IJ, Sperry RJ, eds. *Advances in Anesthesia*. St. Louis, Mo: Mosby-Year Book, Inc.;1995:145.

46 Mercadante S. Pharmacotherapy for breakthrough cancer pain. *Drugs*. 2012;72:181-190.

47 Farrar JT, Cleary J, Rauck R, Busch M, Nordbrock E. Oral transmucosal fentanyl citrate: randomized, double-blinded, placebo-controlled trial for treatment of breakthrough pain in cancer patients. *J Natl Cancer Inst*. 1998;90:611-616.

Chapter 2

What is cancer breakthrough pain?

Definitions

The original definition of cancer breakthrough pain (cBTP), given by Portenoy and Hagen [1], is the template upon which the majority of subsequent definitions have been based: breakthrough pain (BTP) is a transitory increase in pain to greater than moderate intensity on a baseline pain of moderate intensity or less. Other authors have modified this definition in a number of ways but the majority of authors require that the background, baseline, or persistent pain be adequately controlled in-line with the original definition given by Portenoy and Hagen. Similarly, the definition of cBTP used in this text requires adequately controlled baseline pain as well:

> " cBTP is a transient exacerbation of pain that occurs either spontaneously, or in relation to a specific predictable or unpredictable trigger, despite relatively stable and adequately controlled background pain [2,3]. "

Note that by definition, for a particular flare of pain to be cBTP, the patient must have cancer; however, the actual source of the pain may or may not be directly related to the cancer. For example, the pain may be secondary to chemotherapy or other cancer-related treatments, tumor invasion of bone or nerve, a herniated disc, or osteoarthritis [4,5].*

D. R. Taylor., *Managing Cancer Breakthrough Pain*,
DOI: 10.1007/978-1-908517-83-8_2, © Springer Healthcare 2013

Adequate pain control

Twycross has described pain control in the hospice setting and developed the practical concept of "good enough" pain relief [3,6]. Pain relief is "good enough" when the patient can accomplish desired rational goals without undue suffering. It is ideal if complete pain relief can be achieved without unacceptable side effects. However, sometimes cancer pain does not respond completely to analgesics, surgery, nerve blocks, or cancer-directed therapy; in other words, the patient's pain may not be completely eliminated. In these cases, clinicians must seek "good enough" pain relief for the patient. The clinician must help the patient understand what rational goals are based on the patient's current state of health. Adequately controlled pain will usually correspond to a pain score of 0–4 on the Numerical Rating Scale, where 0 represents no pain and 10 represents the worst imaginable pain [7].

Cancer breakthrough pain versus background pain flares

In addition to understanding the concept of "adequate control", it is also imperative that the clinician be able to distinguish cBTP from background pain flares (BGPF). Most authors consider the "breaking through" aspect of cBTP to be the pain overriding the otherwise stable control of the patient's basal or background pain (Figure 2.1A[†]) [8–10]. Persistent pain and cBTP are distinct clinical entities and should be assessed individually [10]. Basal, background, or persistent pain for patients with cBTP usually lasts longer than 12 hours/day and is adequately controlled by an around-the-clock (ATC) analgesic medication, usually an opioid. However, a flare of pain or a BGPF (Figure 2.1B[†]) occurs when the background pain is not under

---

*Some authors have protested creating a separate category for cancer pain and contend that cancer pain should be considered under the categories of either acute or chronic pain. While the discussion of the advantages and disadvantages of defining cancer pain as somehow distinct from other forms of acute or chronic pain will not be expanded upon here, the fact that cancer pain management often blends into palliative care and end-of-life care adds a unique dimension to cancer pain management [5].

[†]When looking at pain versus time diagrams (Figures 2.1A, B), it should be noted that the height of the background pain line reflects the intensity of the pain prior to treatment rather than the actual current pain level. Since, by definition, cBTP requires that the background, persistent pain is adequately controlled all the pain diagrams would show a low-basal pain if the current basal pain were represented; however, this would not add any information to the diagrams. This contrivance of representing the basal-pain level prior to treatment in these diagrams helps give a better picture of

adequate control [2]. In contrast to Figure 2.1A, where the background pain is under adequate control, Figure 2.1B shows poorly controlled, persistent background pain and a flare of pain. Rescue pain medications, generally short-acting opioids (SAOs), are used to treat BGPFs, whereas both SAOs and rapid-onset opioids (ROOs) may be used to treat cBTP.

In a sense, the origin of cBTP management lies in the use of rescue medication as a method of titration of the ATC analgesic. This evolution of cancer pain management and the similarity of cBTP episodes to flares of pain seen in patients without adequately controlled background pain has led to some disagreement in the literature about the terminology of cBTP. Unfortunately, there is not a universally agreed upon terminology for cBTP management [11] and it is not uncommon to see the term "rescue dose" or "rescue medication" and "breakthrough dose" or "breakthrough medication" used interchangeably in the literature [2,8,12]. This can create some confusion. Readers may see the term "rescue dose" applied to a ROO used to treat spontaneous cBTP or see the term "breakthrough dose" used to refer to the use of morphine for titration of the ATC analgesic dose. When reading publications about cBTP, the reader should determine how the terms were defined within the text to establish the author's true meaning.

Differential diagnoses
Intermittent pain or nonbreakthrough pain
A study by Mystakidou et al investigated patients with cancer who did not have background pain but who had intermittent flares of pain [13]. Although this pain is very similar in characteristics to cBTP, as there is

the overall pain state of the patient. If the basal pain is adequately controlled then the basal analgesic line is drawn above the basal pain line (Figure 2.1A). If the basal pain is not adequately controlled then the basal analgesic line is drawn below the basal pain line (Figure 2.1B). It is hoped that these simple pain versus time diagrams can help clinicians and healthcare professionals better conceptualize a framework for managing cancer pain. Constructing a pain versus time diagram may help the clinician determine an appropriate analgesic regimen for a patient. The time intervals are not specified in Figures 2.1A, B because the time interval between cBTP episodes can vary from minutes to hours to days. Rather, in clinical practice it is important to know when the cBTP occurs in relation to other life events. As will be discussed later in the text, the time interval between cBTP episodes is one of the criteria that are used in determining whether it is appropriate to treat each cBTP episode individually or whether the basal analgesic should be increased. This can also help with detecting end-of-dose failure and incident pain.

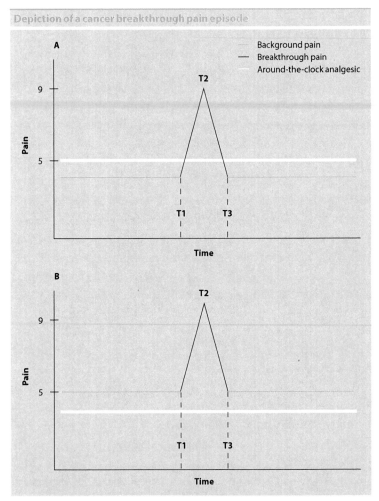

Figure 2.1 Depiction of a cancer breakthrough pain episode. A, Cancer breakthrough pain with stable background pain. The patient's pain is under stable, adequate control (background pain is ≤4 out of 10 on the NRS) since the background pain line is below the around-the-clock analgesic line. At T1, the patient experiences a sudden, rapid increase in pain that "breaks through" the around-the-clock analgesic; this cancer breakthrough pain episode peaks at 9 out of 10 on the NRS at T2; T3 represents how long the breakthrough pain lasts. Note that an analgesic line above the basal pain line does not mean that the basal pain has been reduced to zero but rather that the background pain is adequately controlled (≤4 out of 10 on NRS). **B**, Cancer background pain flare, without adequate control. The patient's pain is not under adequate control since the around-the-clock analgesic line is below the patient's background pain line. At T1, the patient experiences a sudden, rapid increase of pain, which peaks at 9 out of 10 on the NRS (T2) and last until T3. This is known as a background pain flare. NRS, Numerical Rating Scale.

no background pain, it is by definition not cBTP or a BGPF; the authors have instead suggested the names "intermittent pain" or "nonbreakthrough pain" [13]. There are very few studies on nonbreakthrough cancer pain; it is only mentioned here for completeness and so that the practitioner will recognize that while these flares of nonbreakthrough pain may seem like cBTP, they are not.

End-of-dose failure

Some authors have included end-of-dose failure as a form of pseudo-cBTP that occurs when the dosing interval between long-acting agents is longer than the effective duration of the drug [14]. The drug level falls too low before the next dose is administered to provide analgesic coverage and the patient experiences pain [15]. This type of pain is not actually cBTP and is best managed by addressing the frequency or dose of ATC basal analgesic rather than by adding a cBTP medication [16–18]. For this reason, other authors, including myself [2], have not included end-of-dose failure as a form of cBTP [3].

Characteristics of cancer breakthrough pain

Studies show that cBTP occurs in 40–80% of patients with cancer-related pain [19,20]. Thus, its severity and frequency of occurrence underscore the relevance of cBTP treatment in the overall management of cancer pain [21,22]. cBTP is generally of moderate-to-severe intensity, with a rapid onset of 3–15 minutes. Episodes last for approximately 60 minutes (Table 2.1, Figure 2.1A), but can range in duration from 1 to 240 minutes [23]. cBTP episodes occur approximately 3–5 times per day [14,23,24].

Characteristics of cancer breakthrough pain	
Characteristics of cBTP	**Average**
Time-to-peak severity	3–15 minutes
Severity	Moderate to severe
Duration	30–60 minutes
Number of episodes per day	3–5

Table 2.1 Characteristics of cancer breakthrough pain. cBTP is a transitory pain that "breaks through" background or persistent pain, which is adequately controlled by an around-the-clock medication. cBTP, cancer breakthrough pain.

Types of cancer breakthrough pain

There are two main types of cBTP: predictable and spontaneous (idiopathic) or unpredictable (Table 2.2) [3]. Predictable cBTP is most often due to movement and it has an understandable cause. Spontaneous cBTP occurs without warning and is not associated with any particular event or activity. It has no identifiable cause and it does not have a consistent temporal relationship between the cBTP pain episode, basal analgesic dose, or activity. In a multicenter European study involving 320 patients with cancer, 44% of patients reported experiencing incident-related or predictable cBTP, 39% had spontaneous cBTP, and 17% reported having both types of cBTP [24].

Assessment of cancer breakthrough pain

Before initiating treatment for a patient with suspected cBTP, a physician should first confirm that the patient has cancer and the patient's background pain is under adequate control [10]. Once that is confirmed, one of the first steps in assessing cBTP is to educate the patient about the definition of both cBTP and background pain [25]. This educational process will help the patient and physician establish a common language for discussing the patient's pain.

A number of tools have been developed for the assessment of cBTP, but none are currently widely used in clinical practice [8]. Haugen et al [8] reviewed available global literature on the assessment of cBTP and concluded that ideally the clinician should determine:

- the number of cBTP episodes;
- the relationship between cBTP and the background pain (the same or different);
- the intensity of the cBTP episodes;

Type of cancer breakthrough pain	Characteristics
Predictable	Consistent temporal relationship with precipitating factor
Spontaneous (idiopathic) or unpredictable	Not induced by a readily identifiable cause; inconsistent temporal relationship with a precipitating factor

Table 2.2 Types of cancer breakthrough pain. Data from Bennett et al [3].

- the temporal factors of cBTP; including its frequency, onset, duration, and relationship to fixed analgesic dose;
- where cBTP episodes are occurring in the body;
- the quality of the cBTP (eg, burning, aching, lancinating, throbbing);
- any potential treatment-related factors, including exacerbating and relieving factors, such as precipitating events and predictability, response to treatment (time-to-meaningful relief), and treatment satisfaction; and
- whether the cBTP interferes with activities of daily living and quality of life.

An assessment tool is available (see page 20) that incorporates many of these features [3,8]. The topics not specifically covered within the assessment form and deemed important by the clinician can be included during the patient interview or added as additional questions to the tool.

More discussion regarding a practical approach to assessment and diagnosis of patients with suspected cBTP will be further described through case studies in Chapter 4.

Understanding cancer breakthrough pain and its treatment

Once a patient's cBTP has been confirmed and fully assessed, several treatment options may be pursued. First and foremost, since cBTP varies per patient, the treatment must be individualized and tailored to each patient's specific needs (like the World Health Organization recommends "for the individual" and with "attention to detail"). Depending on the patient's cBTP, nonpharmacological methods (eg, heat, ice, distraction, guided imagery, massage, or transcutaneous electrical nerve stimulation [TENS]) [26,27] may be used to manage their cBTP. However, if nonpharmacological approaches are not sufficient, there are a number of pharmacological approaches, specifically ROOs, available based on the varying types, frequencies, durations, and temporal profiles of a patient's cBTP. As ROOs are currently the only medications approved for the treatment of cBTP, this class will be discussed in general terms below, and specific ROOs will be further explored in Chapter 3.

Initial cancer breakthrough pain assessment

Name: Date:

1. Do you have episodes of severe pain or breakthrough pain?

2. Please refer to the diagram (right) to answer the next questions. Is your pain more like Peak 1 (which rapidly peaks in intensity) or Peak 2 (which peaks gradually in intensity overtime)?

   A. How long does the pain last on average?   Peak 1: _____   Peak 2: _____

   B. Do you have some episodes of both Peak 1 and Peak 2?   Yes ☐ No ☐

Answer the following three questions on a scale of 0–10; 0 represents no pain and 10 represents the worst imaginable pain

3. Rate your average background pain over the past 24 hours:

4. Rate your average breakthrough pain intensity over the past 24 hours:

5. Rate the maximum intensity of your breakthrough pain in the past 24 hours:

6. How many breakthrough pain episodes have you had over the past 24 hours?

7. If you have multiple breakthrough pain episodes, how long does each episode of breakthrough pain last?

8. How long is it from the time the pain first occurs to when the pain is at its worst?

9. Where does the breakthrough pain occur? What does it feel like?

   Explain:

10. Is your breakthrough pain the same type of pain as your background pain or is it different?

    Explain:

11. Do you have more than one type of breakthrough pain?   Yes ☐ No ☐

    If yes, explain:

12. Do you have breakthrough pain with specific movements of activities?   Yes ☐ No ☐

    If yes, explain:

13. Does your breakthrough pain occur spontaneously or for no apparent reason?   Yes ☐ No ☐

    If yes, explain:

14. Does your breakthrough pain occur just before you are supposed to take   Yes ☐ No ☐
    your next dose of pain medicine?

    If yes, explain:

15. Does your breakthrough pain have any relation to the time of day?   Yes ☐ No ☐

    If yes, explain:

16. What impact does the breakthrough pain have on your daily activities at home/work? Are you able to do the things you want/need to do?

17. Are there any things that you avoid doing or that you are able to do only with severe pain?

18. What do you do to relieve the breakthrough pain?

19. What types of treatment and/or drugs have you used? How long did you use them? Were they effective? Are they still effective?

    Describe your current breakthrough pain treatment (if any):

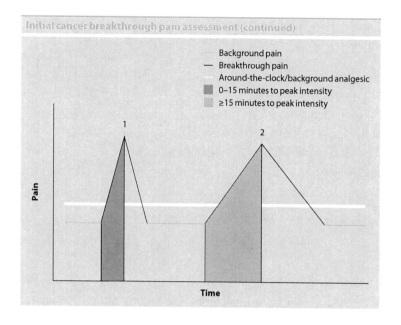

Initial cancer breakthrough pain assessment (continued)

- - - Background pain
—— Breakthrough pain
—— Around-the-clock/background analgesic
■ 0–15 minutes to peak intensity
■ ≥15 minutes to peak intensity

Different types of cancer breakthrough pain episodes in relation to treatment

Cancer breakthrough pain and background pain flares

Understanding the difference between cBTP and BGPF, as described in Figures 2.1A and 2.1B, is critical for determining the pharmacological approach that will be most appropriate for the patient. The dose of medication used for treating a BGPF – know as a "rescue dose" – is usually incorporated into the daily ATC dose for background pain management during dose titration. However, ROOs are titrated to control cBTP and they are not incorporated into the ATC background pain medication since the background pain should already be under adequate control when a ROO is initiated.

High-basal versus low-basal pain

The basal analgesic dose does not predict the cBTP medication dose. A patient with a high-level of basal pain and associated high-basal analgesic dose could have cBTP episodes of mild intensity (Figure 2.2A) [2,24,28,29], which may only require small doses of cBTP medications, or nonpharmacological measures to manage the cBTP episodes. Meanwhile, a patient with low-level basal pain and correspondingly low levels of basal analgesic medication could experience high-intensity cBTP episodes, where high doses of cBTP medications may be more appropriate (Figure 2.2B) [2,24,28,29].

In early studies with oral transmucosal fentanyl citrate (OTFC), the first ROO approved for cBTP in the United States, no relationship was found between the successful dose of OTFC and the total daily dose of ATC opioid, indicating that the optimal dose of OTFC could not be

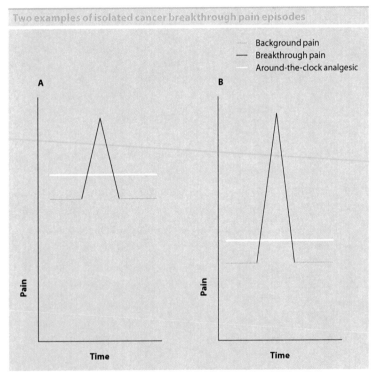

Figure 2.2 Two examples of isolated cancer breakthrough pain episodes. A, The patient has high-level basal pain, requiring a high dose of opioids, while the cBTP episode is of mild intensity and may thus be controlled with a small dose of opioid, and even possibly with nonpharmacological means. **B,** The patient has mild basal pain, but the cBTP episode is of severe intensity and may thus require a high dose of opioid for control. Note: not every cBTP episode requires an opioid for management; not all cBTP episodes are the same, even in the same patient, thus individualization of treatment is mandatory. cBTP, cancer breakthrough pain. Data from Davies et al [2], Davies et al [24], Green et al [28], and Davies et al [29].

predicted by the total daily dose of fixed-schedule opioid for basal pain [14,30]. This led to the recommendation to titrate-to-effect OTFC, starting with the lowest dose and increasing it in a stepwise fashion until cBTP became adequately controlled [31,32]. Similar recommendations have subsequently been made for all of the approved ROOs.

Varying types of cancer breakthrough pain episodes for one patient

Studies have shown that cBTP episodes vary both between individuals and also within individuals [14,24]. In any particular patient, some cBTP episodes may be severe while other episodes may be of minimal intensity. The severe cBTP episodes may require a potent ROO for management, while the less intense episodes might be managed with an SAO or nonpharmacologic techniques, such as heat, ice, distraction, imagery, massage, or TENS [26,27], and, as such, a patient with several types of basal pain and cBTP episodes may therefore require various types of treatment (ie, long-acting opioids [LAO] for basal pain, SAOs, and ROOs). Some physicians may feel uncomfortable with prescribing multiple medications; however, sometimes such treatment plans may be required for optimal results. A physician can tailor the pain management regimen most appropriately for the patient by listening to the patient's needs, the caregiver's input (if applicable), and determining pain patterns and pathophysiology (neuropathic, nociceptive, visceral, and somatic).

Predictable versus spontaneous cancer breakthrough pain and treatment

Predictable and spontaneous cBTP episodes may be managed differently (Table 2.3). Since predictable cBTP has a consistent temporal relationship with an activity, the pain can be preemptively managed with a regular opioid, such as an SAO, taken at least 30–45 minutes prior to the activity that causes the pain [33]. Spontaneous episodes of cBTP require a different approach as these episodes are unpredictable. SAOs have a longer time to onset (30–45 minutes) than ROOs (5–15 minutes), thus ROOs are more appropriate for spontaneous episodes of cBTP (Figure 1.6) [7]. The peak of the analgesic effect with standard opioids, such as oral

Type of cancer breakthrough pain	Treatment
Predictable	Preemptive, SAO 30–45 minutes prior to activity
Spontaneous (idiopathic) or unpredictable	ROO or SAO*

Table 2.3 Treatment guidelines for predictable and spontaneous cancer breakthrough pain. *If the pain escalates slowly to maximum intensity, an SAO may be appropriate. ROO, rapid-onset opioid; SAO, short-acting opioid. Data from Bennett et al [3].

morphine, oxycodone, hydromorphone, or methadone, may occur after the pain has resolved [33,34]. Many drugs, such as nasal morphine [35,36], oral methadone [37], nasal sufentanil [38], and subcutaneous hydromorphone [39], have been studied for the treatment of cBTP; however, to date, the only drugs specifically approved for the treatment of cBTP in the United States or the European Union remain fentanyl-based ROOs.

Duration of cancer breakthrough pain episodes and treatment

The duration and time to peak-pain intensity of cBTP episodes also needs to be taken into account when considering treatment. For example, if a cBTP episode is very rapid in onset and very brief in duration (eg, peak intensity occurs in 3–5 minutes and duration of cBTP is 15–30 minutes) it is reasonable to consider using the ROO with the fastest onset time and the shortest duration of action [40]. If the cBTP episode has a slower onset, then a ROO with a slightly slower onset time might be more appropriate. If the cBTP episode is of long duration, several hours or more, then an SAO might be appropriate. The goal is to try to match the time–intensity profile of the cBTP episode with the action profile of the medication used to treat the episode.

Studies of the duration of effect of cBTP medications are complicated by the fact that most cBTP episodes are expected to last for a relatively short period of time and in any patient, episodes can vary in intensity and the frequency of episodes may not be constant [41]. Thus, it is not possible to tell if a cBTP episode was suppressed by an analgesic or if it naturally resolved before the analgesic wore off. For this reason most cBTP studies do not report on the duration of action of the drugs. Nonetheless, duration of ROOs can be judged based on their means of absorption into the body (eg, oral, additional gastrointestinal absorption, nasal, etc). This will be further discussed in Chapter 3.

Physicians must also take into account that if a drug has a duration of action significantly beyond the duration of the cBTP episode, the risk of adverse effects, such as sedation or respiratory depression, might increase as the drug's sedative and respiratory depressant effects would not be opposed by the cBTP episode during the latter part of its action [9,33]; acute pain antagonizes the respiratory depressant effect of opioids and stimulates respiration [42]. This is another reason to match the drug's time course of action to the time course of the cBTP [43].

Frequency of cancer breakthrough pain episodes and treatment

The frequency of cBTP episodes has implications for treatment. As a general rule, if the patient consistently requires treatment for more than 4 cBTP episodes per day, then the adequacy of the ATC medication should be reassessed [44]. For example, it is reasonable to treat a patient with 4 cBTP episodes per day with an SAO or ROO, depending upon the temporal profile of the cBTP episodes. In contrast, if a patient has, for example, 11 cBTP episodes per day that occur every 2 hours, then taking medication to compensate for each cBTP episode can become burdensome for the patient or caregiver; it may be more appropriate for the patient to increase the ATC medication (eg, LAO) by titration.

References

1   Portenoy RK, Hagen NA. Breakthrough pain: definition and management. *Oncology (Williston Park)*. 1989;3(8 Suppl):25-29.
2   Davies AN, Dickman A, Reid C, Stevens AM, Zeppetella G; Science Committee of the Association for Palliative Medicine of Great Britain and Ireland. The management of cancer-related breakthrough pain: recommendations of a task group of the Science Committee of the Association for Palliative Medicine of Great Britain and Ireland. *Eur J Pain*. 2009;13:331-338.
3   Bennett D, Burton AW, Fishman S, et al. Consensus panel recommendations for the assessment and management of breakthrough pain: Part 1 Assessment. *P T*. 2005;30:296-301.
4   Turk DC, Okifuji A. Pain terms and taxonomies of pain. In: Fishman SM, Ballantyne JC, Rathmell JP, eds. *Bonica's Management of Pain*. 4th ed. New York, NY: Lippincott Williams & Wilkins; 2010:13-23.
5   Berger AM, Portenoy RK, Weissman DE. Preface. In: Berger A, Portenoy RK, Weissman DE, eds. *Principles and Practice of Supportive Oncology*. Lippincott Williams & Wilkins. Philadelphia, PA; 1998:xix-xx.
6   Twycross RG. Where there is hope, there is life: a view from the hospice. In: Keown J, ed. *Euthanasia Examined: Ethical, Clinical and Legal Perspectives*. New York, NY: Cambridge University Press; 1995:141-168.

7 Mercadante S. Managing breakthrough pain. *Curr Pain Headache Rep*. 2011;15:244-249.

8 Haugen DF, Hjermstad MJ, Hagen N, Caraceni A, Kaasa S; European Palliative Care Research Collaborative (EPCRC). Assessment and classification of cancer breakthrough pain: a systematic literature review. *Pain*. 2010;149:476-482.

9 Zeppetella G. Breakthrough pain in cancer patients. *Clin Oncol (R Coll Radiol)*. 2011;23:393-398.

10 Payne R. Recognition and diagnosis of breakthrough pain. *Pain Med*. 2007;8(8 Suppl 1):S3-S7.

11 Zeppetella G. Impact and management of breakthrough pain in cancer. *Curr Opin Support Palliat Care*. 2009;3:1-6.

12 Mercadante S, Radbruch L, Caraceni A, et al; Steering Committee of the European Association for Palliative Care (EAPC) Research Network. Episodic (breakthrough) pain: consensus conference of an expert working group of the European Association for Palliative Care. *Cancer*. 2002;94:832-839.

13 Bhatnagar S, Upadhyay S, Mishra S. Prevalence and characteristics of breakthrough pain in patients with head and neck cancer: a cross-sectional study. *J Palliat Med*. 2010;13:291-295.

14 Portenoy RK, Payne D, Jacobsen P. Breakthrough pain: characteristics and impact in patients with cancer pain. *Pain*. 1999;81:129-134.

15 Kim DY, Song HS, Ahn JS, et al. The dosing frequency of sustained-release opioids and the prevalence of end-of-dose failure in cancer pain control: a Korean multicenter study. *Supportive Care Cancer*. 2011;19:297-301.

16 Hall LM, O'Lenic K. Treatment strategies to overcome end-of-dose failure with oral and transdermal opioids. *J Pharm Pract*. 2011;25:503-509.

17 Paice JA, Fine PG. Pain at the End of Life. In: Ferrell BR, Coyle N, eds. *Oxford Textbook Of Palliative Nursing*. 2nd ed. New York, NY: Oxford University Press, Inc.; 2006:131-155.

18 Patt RB. Classification of cancer pain and cancer pain syndromes. In: Patt RB, ed. *Cancer Pain*. Philadelphia, PA: J.B. Lippincott Company; 1993:3-22.

19 Caraceni A, Martini C, Zecca E, et al; Working Group of an IASP Task Force on Cancer Pain. Breakthrough pain characteristics and syndromes in patients with cancer pain. An international survey. *Palliat Med*. 2004;18:177-183.

20 Caraceni A, Zecca E, Bonezzi C, et al. Gabapentin for neuropathic cancer pain: a randomized controlled trial from the Gabapentin Cancer Pain Study Group. *J Clin Oncol*. 2004;22:2909-2917.

21 Gatti A, Mediati RD, Reale C, et al. Breakthrough pain in patients referred to pain clinics: the Italian pain network retrospective study. *Adv Ther*. 2012;29:464-472.

22 Caraceni A, Bertetto O, Labianca R, et al; Breakthrough/Episodic Pain Italian Study Group. Episodic (breakthrough) pain prevalence in a population of cancer pain patients. Comparison of clinical diagnoses with the QUDEI--Italian questionnaire for intense episodic pain. *J Pain Symptom Manage*. 2012;43:833-841.

23 Portenoy RK, Hagen NA. Breakthrough pain: definition, prevalence and characteristics. *Pain*. 1990;41:273-281.

24 Davies A, Zeppetella G, Andersen S, et al. Multi-centre European study of breakthrough cancer pain: pain characteristics and patient perceptions of current and potential management strategies. *Eur J Pain*. 2011;15:756-763.

25 Hagen NA, Stiles C, Nekolaichuk C, et al. The Alberta Breakthrough Pain Assessment Tool for cancer patients: a validation study using a delphi process and patient think-aloud interviews. *J Pain Symptom Mange*. 2008;35:136-152.

26 National Cancer Institute. Pain (PDQ®) Health Professional Version. www.cancer.gov/cancertopics/pdq/supportivecare/pain/HealthProfessional/page1. Accessed February 1, 2013.

27 Wee B, Hillier R. Pain control. *Medicine*. 2008;36:67-71.

28 Green CR, Montague L, Hart-Johnson TA. Consistent and breakthrough pain in diverse advanced cancer patients: a longitudinal examination. *J Pain Symptom Manage*. 2009;37:831-847.

29 Davies AN, Vriens J, Kennett A, McTaggart M. An observational study of oncology patients' utilization of breakthrough pain medicine. *J Pain Symptom Manage*. 2008;35:406-411.

30 Christie JM, Simmonds M, Patt R, et al. Dose-titration, multicenter study of oral transmucosal fentanyl citrate for the treatment of breakthrough pain in cancer patients using transdermal fentanyl for persistent pain. *J Clin Oncol*. 1998;16:3238-3245.

31 Actiq [package insert]. Frazer, PA: Cephalon, Inc; 2011.

32 Hagen NA, Fisher K, Victorino C, Farrar JT. A titration strategy is needed to manage breakthrough cancer pain effectively: observations from data pooled from three clinical trials. *J Palliat Med*. 2007;10:47-55.

33 Bennett D, Burton AW, Fishman S, et al. Consensus panel recommendations for the assessment and management of breakthrough pain: Part 2 Management. *P T*. 2005;30:354-361.

34 Zeppetella G. Opioids for cancer breakthrough pain: a pilot study reporting patient assessment of time to meaningful pain relief. *J Pain Symptom Manage*. 2008;35:563-567.

35 Fitzgibbon D, Morgan D, Dockter D, Barry C, Kharasch ED. Initial pharmacokinetic, safety and efficacy evaluation of nasal morphine gluconate for breakthrough pain in cancer patients. *Pain*. 2003;106:309-315.

36 Pavis H, Wilcock A, Edgecombe J, et al. Pilot study of nasal morphine-chitosan for the relief of breakthrough pain in patients with cancer. *J Pain Symptom Manage*. 2002;24:598-602.

37 Fisher K, Stiles C, Hagen NA. Characterization of the early pharmacodynamic profile of oral methadone for cancer-related breakthrough pain: a pilot study. *J Pain Symptom Manage*. 2004;28:619-625.

38 Jackson K, Ashby M, Keech, J. Pilot dose finding study of intranasal sufentanil for breakthrough and incident cancer-associated pain. *J Pain Symptom Manage*. 2002;23:450-452.

39 Enting RH, Mucchiano C, Oldenmenger WH, et al. The "pain pen" for breakthrough cancer pain: a promising treatment. *J Pain Symptom Manage*. 2005;29:213-217.

40 Mercadante S, Villari P, Ferrera P, Casuccio A. Optimization of opioid therapy for preventing incident pain associated with bone metastases. *J Pain Symptom Manage*. 2004;28:505-510.

41 Zeppetella G, O'Doherty CA, Collins S. Prevalence and characteristics of breakthrough pain in cancer patients admitted to a hospice. *J Pain Symptom Manage*. 2000;20:87-92.

42 Borgbjerg FM, Nielsen K, Franks J. Experimental pain stimulates respiration and attenuates morphine-induced respiratory depression: a controlled study in human volunteers. *Pain*. 1996;64:123-128.

43 DuBose RA, Berde CB. Respiratory effects of opioids. *IASP Newsletter*. 1997;July/August:1-6.

44 Fine PG, Narayana A, Passik SD. Treatment of breakthrough pain with fentanyl buccal tablet in opioid-tolerant patients with chronic pain: appropriate patient selection and management. *Pain Med*. 2010;11:1024-1036.

Chapter 3

Medications for cancer breakthrough pain

Introduction to rapid-onset opioids

Currently, all the rapid-onset opioids (ROO) approved for treating cancer breakthrough pain (cBTP) in the United States and the European Union are fentanyl-based. Fentanyl is a potent highly lipid-soluble pure μ-agonist first synthesized in the 1950s and introduced into clinical practice in the 1960s. Pharmacological effects of opioid agonists, such as fentanyl, include anxiolysis, euphoria, relaxation, respiratory depression, cough suppression, constipation, miosis, and analgesia [1,2]. It was initially used by anesthesiologists in the operating room as a component of general anesthetics [3]. There the drug remained until the 1980s when researchers observed that such a highly lipid-soluble drug might be delivered through the skin [4]. This led to the development of the first transdermal fentanyl patch in 1990 [5].

More recently, the high-lipid solubility and potency of fentanyl led to the development of the ROO, where the drug is delivered across the buccal, sublingual, or nasal mucosa [6]. The portion of drug directly absorbed across the oral or nasal mucosa then enters into the submucosal capillaries, which avoids first-pass metabolism in the liver and increases the bioavailability of the drug [7]. Transmucosal fentanyl agents are particularly useful for treating cBTP because of their *efficacy*, rather than their *potency*, due to their speed of onset and because their *duration of action* matches the time course of the average cBTP episode (Table 3.1) [1,8–15].

D. R. Taylor., *Managing Cancer Breakthrough Pain*,
DOI: 10.1007/978-1-908517-83-8_3, © Springer Healthcare 2013

Approved rapid-onset opioids

Drug	Formulation	Doses (µg)
ACTIQ® (US) (fentanyl citrate) oral transmucosal lozenge (OTFC)	transmucosal buccal lozenge on a stick	200, 400, 600, 800, 1200, 1600
FENTORA® (US) (fentanyl citrate) buccal tablet (FBT) Effentora® (EU) buccal tablet Fentanyl	buccal tablet with OraVescent® technology	100, 200, 400, 600, 800
ABSTRAL® (US) (fentanyl) sublingual tablet (FST)	sublingual tablet	100, 200, 300, 400, 600, 800
Lazanda® (US) (fentanyl) nasal spray PecFent® (EU) fentanyl pectin nasal spray (FPNS)	pectin-based nasal spray	100, 400
ONSOLIS® (US) fentanyl buccal soluble film (FBSF)	buccal film with BioErodible MucoAdhesive (BEMA™) delivery technology	200, 400, 600, 800, 1200
SUBSYS™ (US) fentanyl sublingual spray (FSS)	sublingual spray-63.6% ethanol	100, 200, 400, 600, 800, 1200[†], 1600[†]
INSTANYL® (EU) intranasal fentanyl spray (INFS)	nasal spray	50, 100, 200

Table 3.1 Approved rapid-onset opioids. *Packaging varies to meet the needs of each patient's specific titration level; for more information on titration schemes, please see appropriate prescribing information per agent and the titration descriptions in the text (page numbers are listed in this table's index column); †Subsys is approved for use at 1200 µg and 1600 µg by combining lower doses (2 x 600 µg, 2 x 800 µg, respectively) to achieve these higher doses. Data from Actiq [package insert] [1], Abstral [package insert] [8], Fentora [package insert] [9], Effentora [package insert] [10], Instanyl [package insert] [11], Lazanda [package insert] [12], PecFent [package insert] [13], Onsolis [package insert] [14], Subsys [package insert] [15].

Packaging*	Generic form available	Index, page number
1 lozenge per blister package, 30 blister packages per shelf carton	Yes	OTFC, general information, 41 OTFC, titration, 43 OTFC, other opioids, 43
4 tablets per blister card, 7 blister cards per pack	Yes	FBT, general information, 44 FBT, titration, 47 FBT, comparative clinical trials, 47
100–400-µg doses in individually sealed blister packages, 12 or 32 tablets per package; 600- and 800-µg doses in individually sealed blister packages, 32 tablets per package	No	FST, general information, 48 FST, titration, 50 FST, other rapid-onset opioids, 50
8 100- or 400-µL sprays per 5.3-mL bottle, 1 or 4 bottles per carton	No	FPNS, general information, 50 FPNS, titration, 52 FPNS, other rapid-onset opioids, 53 FPNS, comparative clinical trials, 53
1 film per protective foil package, 30 foil packages per carton	No	FBSF, general information, 54 FBSF, titration, 56 FBSF, other rapid-onset opioids, 56
1 disposal bottle† per blister package, 6, 14, or 28 blister packages per carton	No	FSS, general information, 57 FSS, titration, 58 FSS, comparative clinical trials, 58
50-, 100-, and 200-µg doses in packs of 2, 6, 8, and 10 containers; also available in same strength multidose vials, 10 or 20 doses per vial	No	INFS, general information, 59 INFS, titration, 59 INFS, OTFC, 59

Transmucosal drugs have a more rapid onset of action than that seen with regular absorption from the gastrointestinal tract [7,16]. Fentanyl achieves equilibrium across the blood–brain barrier in approximately 6 minutes [17], and the rapid onset of the ROOs is primarily due to their lipid solubility and rapid absorption across mucosal membranes and subsequent rapid crossing of the blood–brain barrier. With transmucosal delivery, some of the drug is swallowed and "late" absorption in the gastrointestinal tract occurs, prolonging its duration of action [16]. Manufacturers have tried to further enhance absorption by modifying the drug delivery systems of their respective ROO (Table 3.2) [18], and subsequently the current ROOs are more likely to distinguish themselves from one another by their mode of delivery than by their speed of onset.

Duration of effect

As mentioned in Chapter 2, the duration of effect of cBTP medications in patients with cancer is not known. The unpredictability of cBTP makes

Drug	Drug-delivery system	Result
OTFC	Incorporates nanoparticle technology	Nanoparticle technology maximizes drug–mucosal interactions and increases bioavailability of fentanyl due to high surface area-to-volume ratios of nanosized drug [18]
FBT	Absorption occurs through the buccal mucosa with increased bioavailability. FBT uses OraVescent drug-delivery technology, which employs a chemical reaction to change the pH in the microenvironment of the tablet, increasing the amount of nonionic drug, thus enhancing absorption	Rapid rise of fentanyl in blood level due to increased bioavailability [19,20]
FSS	Increased amount of nonionic fentanyl in sublingual spray; nonionic form of fentanyl is more soluble than its ionic form	Produces reduction in pain intensity in 5 minutes [21]
FPNS	Absorption occurs through the nasal mucosa. FPNS uses a formulation that gels upon contact with the nasal mucosa, thus preventing run-off into the pharynx	Onset of pain relief begins within 5 minutes of administration [22]

Various drug delivery systems of rapid-onset opioids

Table 3.2 Various drug delivery systems of rapid-onset opioids. FBT, fentanyl buccal tablet; FPNS, fentanyl pectin nasal spray; FSS, fentanyl sublingual spray; OTFC, oral transmucosal fentanyl citrate. Data from Csaba et al [18], Durfee et al [19], Darwish et al [20], Rauck et al [21], Taylor et al [22].

determining the duration of effect of an analgesic impossible in the setting of cBTP; a ROO may be affecting the patient or the cBTP episode could just be ending.

Titration

Currently, all ROOs include titration instructions in their package inserts that recommend starting all patients on the lowest dose of the drug and proceeding with a stepwise upward titration. The goal of titration for each patient should be to achieve adequate analgesia with minimal adverse effects [23–25]. Titration schedules vary from one product to another; therefore, it is important to check the package insert for each product to determine the recommended titration protocol prior to use. As none of the ROOs are bioequivalent, patients switching from one transmucosal formulation to another may require repeat titration of the new product [23].

Physicians are recommended to reassure their patients to not be discouraged during the titration process, which may take longer than anticipated, and to keep an open-line of communication with the patient so they may manage their cBTP as effectively as possible. For example, a recent survey of 50 hospice patients with cancer receiving a mean daily oral morphine dose of 132 mg for basal analgesia found that, after dose titration, patients required a mean 800-μg dose of oral transmucosal fentanyl citrate (OTFC) for cBTP after dose titration [26]. In a multicenter study evaluating the use of fentanyl sublingual tablet (FST) for the treatment of cBTP in 131 opioid-tolerant patients with cancer, patients on around-the-clock (ATC) opioids equivalent to 60–1000 mg/day of oral morphine or 50–300 μg/hour of transdermal fentanyl were titrated to effect with FST for their cBTP. The study yielded an effective dose range of 100–800 μg FST, with a median effective dose of 600 μg [27]. It was regularly found in these studies that patients were titrated toward the higher end of the dose spectrum for these drugs, which is not uncommon. Finding the appropriate cBTP management plan for the patient during titration of a ROO is achieved by pain assessment, reassessment, good communication with the patient and/or caregiver, expectation management (providing realistic expectations for pain relief), and reassurance that pain relief is being aggressively pursued [23].

Titrate to effect

Based on the author's extensive clinical experience, titration is a key method in the appropriate use of ROOs for managing a patient's cBTP. A suggested titration scheme can be found in Figure 3.1; however, the prescribing clinician should always refer to a ROO's specific package insert for explicit titration schemes.

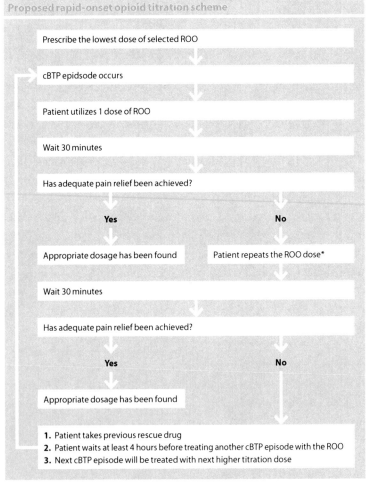

Figure 3.1 Proposed rapid-onset opioid titration scheme. The titration recommendation is based on the author's clinical experience. *Lazanda and Onsolis should be used only once per cBTP episode. cBTP, cancer breakthrough pain; ROO, rapid-onset opioid.

Based on clinical observations while prescribing ROOs, this author recommends that:

1. The titration process must be explained clearly to the patient in terms they understand.
2. Frequent communication with the patient during the titration period by a nurse or clinician can help ensure a successful outcome.
3. Some patients will become disheartened if the first or second ROO dose is not effective. They may think the medication does not work since they may not fully understand the titration process. These patients need to be encouraged to stay on course and to use their rescue medications.
4. If the cBTP is severe and there are no adverse events from the ROO, the clinician may titrate upward every 4 hours.
5. The clinician should know their patient's medical history and preferences to determine appropriate titration recommendations based on their needs. Some patients should talk with a nurse or the clinician prior to each titration step.

As noted in Figure 3.1, it is recommended that most patients start on the lowest dose of most ROOs. The dose is then titrated upward until adequate cBTP relief is obtained. Since the ROOs work rapidly and have a short duration of action, titration can be accomplished quickly, usually within 24–72 hours. If the patient does not obtain significant relief in 30 minutes, generally they may repeat the same dose based on the instructions from their physician, with the exception of fentanyl pectin nasal spray (FPNS) and fentanyl buccal soluble film (FBSF), which should only be dosed once per cBTP episode, per package insert [12–14]. Good communication between the clinician and patient will help to enhance safety and optimize dose titration. For example, it is critically important that the patient understands that they are not to take more than 2 doses per cBTP episode in order to reduce the risk of overdose. Some patients achieve better outcomes if they are required to speak with a nurse or physician prior to taking the second dose.

If the patient still does not achieve adequate relief, they can then use the rescue medication they were originally prescribed prior to starting the ROO. They must then wait 4 hours before resuming the titration; in 4 hours they should treat their next cBTP with the next highest dose. Most patients will achieve an adequate dose with one unit of a particular ROO, but some patients may require the use of 2 or more units at once [28].

It is important to manage the expectations of patients during the ROO titration period. Patients should be informed how and why titration is being started; for example, they should understand that it is being started at the lowest dose of the ROO for safety. The clinician should actively reassure their patient that they will find the dose that provides the best pain relief with the fewest adverse events.

Titration of rapid-onset opioids and high around-the-clock analgesic doses

As mentioned above, titrating ROO doses from the lowest dose upward until effect is generally recommended in all ROO package inserts, and is the safest titration method when initiating treatment. Recently, however, its appropriateness in patients receiving high basal opioid analgesic doses has been questioned [29]. Initial studies with ROOs showed a lack of correlation between the background analgesic dose and the dose of the ROO needed to control the cBTP episodes [30,31]; yet, later observations from pooled data suggested a statistically significant relationship between the cBTP medication dose and the ATC basal analgesic dose [32]. At this time there are not enough data to allow one to recommend the more controversial approach of starting patients on doses of ROO that are proportional to the ATC dose. Clinical experience suggests that highly opioid-tolerant patients are likely to require higher doses of cBTP medication than patients on low doses of opioids [28].

Frequency of dosing

Once an adequate cBTP dose is found, the next step is to determine how often the dose may be repeated in a day. Ideally, the patient's pain should be controlled to the point that they are only experiencing 1–4 cBTP episodes per day [33]. There are no hard "rules" that govern frequency of cBTP dosing; however, very frequent dosing would seem little different than increasing the ATC medication and might add to the "burden of care" for the patient or caregiver. In the final analysis, treatment should be guided by the principles of "for the individual" and "with attention to detail".

The goal is to balance analgesia against side effects. While considering treatment plans for the patient with cBTP, increasing the ATC pain medication to control all the patients pain is sometimes successful. One study of 25 patients with metastatic bone disease and movement-related breakthrough pain showed that increasing the basal analgesic beyond the dose required to adequately manage background pain produced a reduction in the level of incident pain to acceptable levels; however, some patients developed adverse events with this approach that required opioid dose reductions to balance the movement-associated pain intensity with the adverse events [34]. As was seen in this study, increasing the ATC medication to control both basal and breakthrough pain can result in unwanted side effects. Thus, treatment for cBTP episodes should always be individualized and tailored to appropriately control each patient's pain while minimizing side effects. It is important to engage the patient in dialogue about their pain and then listen; the clinician can then develop the optimal treatment plan for the patient.

Considerations for selecting a rapid-onset opioid

Clinicians should be aware of a variety of factors before selecting a ROO, including systemic and localized adverse events, as well as drug–drug interactions.

Rapid-onset opioids and adverse events

Since all ROOs are fentanyl-based, systemic side effects are expected to be similar for all ROOs; however, some ROOs have local effects as well (eg, fentanyl buccal tablets [FBT] may produce mucosal ulceration). Clinicians should always refer to each drug's specific package insert and warnings to review what side effects can apply to their patients. The systemic side effects seen with ROOs are typical of the opioid-drug class, including nausea, vomiting, dizziness, sedation, somnolence, headache, fatigue, asthenia, constipation, dry mouth, and respiratory depression and respiratory arrest [1,8–15,22,35,36].

Rapid-onset opioids and oral mucositis

Patients receiving treatment for cancer may develop oral mucositis (ie, inflammation and ulceration of the oral mucosa) from chemotherapy or radiation; developing oral mucositis is nearly universal in patients receiving radiation for head and neck cancers [37]. Considerations of comorbidities, such as oral mucositis, may guide the practitioner's choice of agents to treat cBTP. For example, some ROOs will require direct application into the buccal cavity (eg, OFTC) or are ethanol-based (eg, fentanyl sublingual spray [FSS]), which may cause irritation and pain for patients with oral mucositis, and will thus not be the optimal choice for that patient.

CYP3A4 inhibitors

Fentanyl is primarily metabolized in the liver predominately by the cytochrome P450 3A4 (CYP3A4) system [38]. The major metabolite is produced by N-dealkylation of fentanyl to norfentanyl by the CYP3A4 system [39]. Interactions may therefore occur when fentanyl is given concurrently with agents that alter the function of CYP3A4. CYP3A4 inhibitors have been shown to increase fentanyl levels and although data on the effects of CYP3A4 induction are more limited, diminished fentanyl concentrations have been seen [40]. All fentanyl-based delivery systems come with a "black box warning" about the potential for overdose if administered with CYP3A4 inhibitors [40]. Inhibitors of the CYP3A4 enzyme include amiodarone, cyclosporine, diazepam, hydroxyzine, quinine, serotonin reuptake inhibitors, indinavir, nelfinavir, ritonavir, clarithromycin, itraconazole, ketoconazole, nefazodone, saquinavir, telithromycin, aprepitant, diltiazem, erythromycin, fluconazole, grapefruit juice, venlafaxine, verapamil, and cimetidine. Consumption of one of these agents by patients on a fentanyl product could cause an increase in fentanyl plasma concentrations, which could potentially result in fatal respiratory depression [41].

The use of CYP3A4 inducers may cause a decrease in fentanyl levels and effect [40]. If the patient is on a fentanyl-based drug, adding an inducer of the CYP34A enzyme might cause a decrease in fentanyl-plasma concentrations, which could cause a deterioration in pain control. Patients concurrently taking fentanyl and a CYP3A4 inducer who subsequently discontinue or reduce the dose of the CYP3A4 inducer might experience an increased fentanyl effect [41]. As such, inducers of the CYP3A4 enzyme, such as barbiturates, carbamazepine, efavirenz, glucocorticoids, modafinil, nevirapine, oxcarbazepine, phenobarbital, phenytoin, pioglitazone, rifabutin, rifampin, St. John's wort, or troglitazone need to be administered or discontinued with caution when prescribing a ROO.

These interactions are more important for drugs that undergo first-pass metabolism in the liver. As a significant portion of all the ROOs is absorbed directly into the blood via the mucosal membranes they may be less affected by CYP3A4 inducers and inhibitors [42].

Bioavailability and dose conversions

Due to differing bioavailability between the ROO formulations, ROOs are not bioequivalent and it is not recommended that clinicians make direct dose conversions between ROOs [43]. The various delivery systems impart different maximum concentrations and bioavailabilities; thus, it is recommended that when switching from one ROO to another, the new drug should be titrated from the lowest dose just as it was done for the initial ROO. This is an important safety point and remembering it will help prevent overdosing or underdosing patients when switching between ROOs.

Opioid tolerance

All ROOs have labeling in their package insert requiring that patients on ROOs be opioid tolerant. As per US Food and Drug Administration (FDA) criteria, patients considered opioid tolerant are those who are taking ATC medicine consisting of at least 60 mg of oral morphine daily, at least 25 µg of transdermal fentanyl per hour, at least 30 mg of oral oxycodone daily, at least 8 mg of oral hydromorphone daily, at least 25 mg oral oxymorphone daily, or an equianalgesic dose of another opioid daily for 1 week or longer (Table 3.3) [44]. Patients entering all of the ROO cBTP studies submitted to regulatory bodies in the United States or the European Union for drug approval had to be on an ATC opioid at

US Food and Drug Administration criteria for opioid tolerance	
Drug	**Daily dose for 1 week**
Morphine	60 mg
Transdermal fentanyl	25 µg/hour
Oxycodone	30 mg
Hydromorphone	8 mg
Oxymorphone	25 mg

Table 3.3 US Food and Drug Administration criteria for opioid tolerance. Patients are considered opioid tolerant if they have been taking the above medications at the indicated dose for *1 week or longer*. They may also have been on any other opioid for 1 week or longer at an equivalent dose of morphine 60 mg/day. Data from Actiq [package insert] [1], Abstral [package insert] [8], Fentora [package insert] [9], Effentora [package insert] [10], Instanyl [package insert] [11], Lazanda [package insert] [12], PecFent [package insert] [13], Onsolis [package insert] [14], Subsys [package insert] [15].

a dose equivalent to or greater than 60 mg morphine for 1 week prior to study entry [1,8–15,35,45–50].

This also indicates that the risk of using ROOs in patients not tolerant to opioids is not well known. There has been some work done using the prototypical ROO, OTFC, in patients not tolerant to opioids with non-cancer pain [43,51,52]; however, while there are some data from this patient population, it is limited, and ROOs are currently only approved for treating BTP in opioid-tolerant patients with cancer.

Additionally, concern has been raised whether patients receiving high doses of opioids for basal analgesia will be good candidates for titration, starting with lowest doses of ROO. The issue is that these patients on high doses of background analgesics are highly opioid tolerant and will likely need high ROO doses; starting titration from the lowest ROO dose might be time consuming and frustrating for the patient. It has been suggested that the clinician could start titration with a relatively higher dose of a ROO in highly opioid-tolerant patients rather than starting from the lowest ROO dose [29]; appropriate package insert and the latest published clinical trial data should be reviewed before pursuing this option.

Rapid-onset opioids

See Table 3.1 for a comprehensive list of all ROOs currently approved in the United States and the European Union.

Oral transmucosal fentanyl citrate

OTFC is formulated as a solid, drug matrix (lozenge) on a handle with white to off-white coloring (Figure 3.2). The drug matrix is designed to dissolve slowly in the mouth to facilitate transmucosal delivery of fentanyl. The handle should be used to place the OTFC unit in the mouth between the cheek and lower gum, and so the patient can move the drug matrix from one side of their mouth to the other for "painting" the unit on the buccal mucosa. The patient is instructed to "twirl the handle often" [1] and to move the medicine at the end of the unit around the mouth, especially along the inside of the cheeks [1], to optimize medication delivery. Because of the amount of patient-dependent activity involved with the use of OTFC, some patients may prefer more passive, less patient-dependent delivery systems [53]. The handle also allows the OTFC unit to be removed from the mouth if signs of excessive opioid effects appear during administration [1].

Since OTFC requires that the unit be rubbed, painted, or twirled against the buccal surface for optimal absorption, OTFC may be painful for patients with oral mucositis. One study found that OTFC might be safe and well-tolerated for patients with grade 3 or 4 radiation-induced oral mucositis; however, some patients did report a burning sensation in

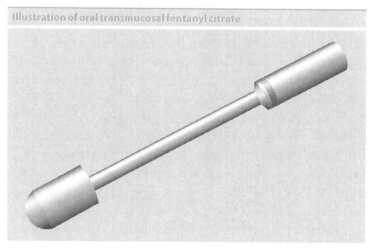

Illustration of oral transmucosal fentanyl citrate

Figure 3.2 Illustration of oral transmucosal fentanyl citrate. Oral transmucosal fentanyl citrate is a solid, white drug matrix (lozenge) on a handle.

the mouth with OTFC [54]. The clinician must engage with their patient to determine if OTFC may become too painful or uncomfortable if their patient has oral mucositis.

The OTFC unit should not be chewed. If OTFC, is chewed and swallowed, this might result in lower peak concentrations and lower bioavailability than when consumed as intended [1]. Also, based on clinical experience, this author has found that the design of OTFC may prompt some patients to suck on the unit much like a lollipop; sucking on the unit with it held between the tongue and roof of the mouth leads to suboptimal absorption of the fentanyl and reduced clinical effect. Also, although early reports on OTFC described the drug as a lollipop [55], one might consider avoiding terms such as "fentanyl lollipop" as children might misconstrue the drug to be candy if they hear it referred to in such terms. Ironically, confectioner's sugar forms one of the inactive ingredients of OTFC; each unit contains about 2 grams of sugar [56]. This is part of the "edible glue" that holds the lozenge together and undoubtedly helps mask the bitterness of the fentanyl [1], and it is this confectioner's sugar that is thought to contribute to the dental caries sometimes seen with the use of this drug [57,58]. The occurrence of dry mouth associated with the use of opioid medications (such as fentanyl) may add to this risk. Postmarketing reports of dental decay have been received in patients taking OTFC. In some of these patients, dental decay occurred despite reported routine oral hygiene. As dental decay in patients with cancer may be multifactorial, it is recommended that patients using OTFC should consult their dentist to ensure appropriate oral hygiene [1]. OTFC, however, may not be the appropriate ROO for patients who may not have good dental hygiene.

Some moisture is required for the OTFC unit to dissolve. If the patient suffers from dry mouth, this may need to be treated with a sialagogue or by having the patient moisten their mouth with water prior to administering the OTFC. The lozenge can be gently rubbed against the buccal mucosa or the unit can be placed in the buccal gutter between the cheek and lower gum. It should be moved from side to side occasionally to help ensure that the unit stays moist. If severe dry mouth is a problem, the unit can be dipped in water when the unit is switched from side to side.

With OTFC, approximately 25% of fentanyl is absorbed via the buccal mucosa while the remaining 75% is absorbed by swallowing. The overall bioavailability of OTFC is approximately 50% [1,59] The medium time to maximum plasma concentration is approximately 20–40 minutes [16]. Many patients report a significant improvement in their pain within 15 minutes of administering OTFC [60] and OTFC has been found to work faster to relieve cBTP than morphine, oxycodone, hydromorphone, and methadone [26].

Oral transmucosal fentanyl citrate and titration

Like all ROOs, it is recommended that titration of OTFC to control cBTP start with the lowest dose. The unit's strength is marked on the individual solid-drug matrix and the handle tag. OTFC is available in microgram doses of 200, 400, 600, 800, 1200, and 1600 [1]. There are a wide variety of OTFC dosage forms available, allowing 74% of patients involved in clinical studies to titrate to an appropriate dose [61]. The process of drug consumption should take about 15 minutes for optimal drug absorption. Please see package insert for further information on titration of OTFC [1].

In one study determining the efficacy of OTFC versus placebo, there was a tendency for patients who were on higher doses of regular-release rescue medication to generally require larger doses of OTFC; however, this relationship was not strong enough to allow for the calculation of a conversion factor. It was postulated that the weak correlation of previous rescue dose to OTFC dose might be due to changes in the pharmacodynamics of treatment when a rapidly absorbed drug, such as transmucosal fentanyl, is used [31]. Early studies found no correlation between the ATC background analgesic dose and titrated OTFC dose [49,62]; however, subsequent studies have suggested that there may be a correlation between ATC background-pain dose and OTFC dose [63].

Oral transmucosal fentanyl citrate and other opioids

In a study directly comparing OTFC to oral morphine for reducing cBTP intensity, OTFC was found more efficacious than morphine [64]. OTFC has linear pharmacokinetics (eg, 200 µg + 200 µg = 400 µg) [65].

In the postoperative setting, 200 µg OTFC was shown to be equivalent to 2 mg intravenous morphine, and 800 µg OTFC was equivalent to 8 mg intravenous morphine [66,67]. The fact that the clinician can achieve analgesia with an oral agent as quickly as with intravenous morphine represents a dramatic advancement in pain management. If the patient does not already have intravenous access established at the time of need, using OTFC would be expected to be faster than establishing an intravenous line and then administering intravenous morphine. Such a situation might arise in trauma care; for example, the use of OTFC has been reported for pain management in combat casualties [68].

Fentanyl buccal tablet

FBT is supplied in cartons containing 7 blister cards with 4 white tablets in each card. Patients must be cautioned not to attempt to push the pills through the covering as the child-resistant nature of the packaging prevents accessing the tablets in this manner and the pills may be crushed and rendered unusable. FBT is recommended to be applied between the cheek and gum above the rear molar (Figure 3.3A); the sublingual and buccal routes of administration have been shown to be bioequivalent [69,70]. FBT utilizes the OraVescent® drug-delivery technology, which generates a chemical reaction when the tablet comes in contact with saliva (Figure 3.3B) [71]. Citric acid and sodium bicarbonate are incorporated into the tablet, and when these make contact with the water in saliva they react to release carbon dioxide. The combination of carbon dioxide and water forms carbonic acid, which produces an initial fall in pH and improves dissolution of the tablet. The carbonic acid then dissociates into carbon dioxide and water, and effervesces into the atmosphere; the pH rises, increasing membrane permeation of the fentanyl. The increase in pH causes some of the ionized fentanyl to convert to the nonionized form, which is more permeable to cell membranes and this can result in more rapid absorption [45,71]. Thus, it is believed that the transient pH changes accompanying the OraVescent reaction may optimize dissolution of the tablet (at a lower pH) and membrane penetration of fentanyl across the buccal mucosa (at a higher pH) [71].

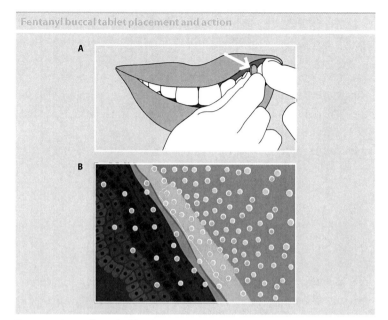

Figure 3.3 Fentanyl buccal tablet placement and action. A, patients are to place a fentanyl buccal tablet in the mouth above a rear molar tooth between the upper cheek and gum.
B, The tablet is to be left in place until it dissolves [9]. Adapted from Fentora [package insert] [9], Breakthroughcancerpain.org [72].

FBT must be left in place for 14–25 minutes until the tablet is dissolved [9], The FBT does not generally require water for administration as it is not swallowed, but it does require saliva or a moistened mucous membrane for the effervescent reaction to take place. If a patient has an extremely dry mouth, the author has found that treatment with a sialagogue or having the patient swish water in their mouth will often solve this problem. In some patients, the tablet may persist for a longer period of time; however, studies have shown that most of the active ingredient, fentanyl, is gone from the tablet after 20 minutes and that a prolonged "dwell time" (ie, the length of time of the FBT is retained in the buccal cavity) does not alter drug absorption [73]; analysis of the effect of dwell time on the pharmacokinetics of FBT revealed a mean buccal dwell time of 14–25 minutes (range: 3–62 minutes) [69,73]. Thus, after 30 minutes, patients should be instructed to swallow any remaining tablet with water [9,74].

Following buccal administration of FBT, fentanyl is readily absorbed with an absolute bioavailability of 65%. The pharmacokinetic profile is largely the result of an initial absorption from the buccal mucosa, with venous peak plasma concentrations generally attained within an hour after administration. Approximately 50% of the total administered dose is absorbed transmucosally and becomes systemically available. The remaining half of the total dose is swallowed and undergoes more prolonged absorption from the gastrointestinal tract [75]. Sublingual and buccal administration produce equivalent results [69,70].

FBT has been shown to have linear pharmacokinetics from 100 μg to 1300 μg [69,76]. However, one study reported that while total systemic exposure increased in a dose-proportional manner with FBT doses of 270–1300 μg, doses above 810 μg showed a less than linear increase in maximum concentration [77]. Thus, at higher doses than are commonly used, the total absorption of FBT is linear but the maximum concentration of drug is not strictly linear. Since the drug is titrated to effect, this is unlikely to have a significant impact on clinical practice.

The use of FBT may result in application site reactions [9]. In clinical trials, 10% of all patients exposed to FBT reported reactions at the site of application. These reactions ranged from paresthesia to ulceration and bleeding. Application site reactions occurring in ≥1% of patients were pain (4%), ulcer (3%), and irritation (3%). Application site reactions tended to occur early in treatment, were self-limited, and only resulted in treatment discontinuation for 2% of patients [9].

The chemical reaction of FBT produces a fall in pH in the microenvironment around the tablet and some patients with oral mucositis find the "acid phase" (low pH) painful and do not tolerate FBT well. This chemical reaction may also contribute to the mucosal ulcers that are sometimes seen with this preparation. In one clinical trial of FBT, 2% of patients withdrew from the study because of application site ulcers [54]. Another trial found that the absorption profile of FBT (>200 μg) was similar in patients with oral mucositis (>grade 2) or without oral mucositis, which suggests that dose adjustment of FBT is not required when mild oral mucositis is present [77,78].

Fentanyl buccal tablets and titration

FBT comes in the following microgram doses: 100, 200, 400, 600, and 800. To manage cBTP episodes, it is recommended that titration of FBT start with the lowest dose followed by upward titration; however, for patients being converted from OTFC to FBT prescribers should review the FBT package insert table to find the appropriate starting titration dose (Table 3.4) [9,10]. The bioavailability of FBT is higher than OTFC [20]; thus, for a given dose of OTFC, a reduction of approximately 30% is needed to convert it to FBT. A 1 : 1 conversion of OTFC : FBT could result in an overdose [9].

Fentanyl buccal tablet and comparative clinical trials

FBT has been shown to be effective for cBTP in a number of placebo-controlled studies [45,79–81]. One study (N=125) showed greater reduction of pain intensity of cBTP episodes in 10 minutes with FBT compared to placebo ($P<0.0001$) [82]. When compared to the first ROO (OTFC), FBT has been shown to deliver a larger proportion of the fentanyl dose transmucosally and produce a greater early systemic exposure [25,83]. FBT has a higher absolute bioavailability (65%) compared to OTFC (47%) [74]. More fentanyl is absorbed transmucosally from FBT than OTFC (48% versus 22%), and median time-to-maximum serum concentration is shorter for FBT (47 minutes) than OTFC (91 minutes) [74]. The extent of

Current OTFC dose (µg)	Starting FBT dose
200	100-µg tablet
400	100-µg tablet
600	200-µg tablet
800	200-µg tablet
1200	2 x 200-µg tablet
1600	2 x 200-µg tablet

Appropriate starting titration recommendations for FBT when patient were previously prescribed OTFC

Table 3.4 Appropriate starting titration recommendations for FBT when patient were previously prescribed OTFC. The doses of FBT in this table are starting doses for initiating titration and are not intended to represent equianalgesic doses to OTFC. FBT, fentanyl buccal tablets; OTFC, oral transmucosal fentanyl citrate. Adapted from Fentora [package insert] [9], Effentora [package insert] [10].

fentanyl absorption is greater following administration of FBT compared to OTFC by about 30% [20]. Thus, FBT cannot be substituted for OTFC on a µg for µg basis, which could result in an overdose [74]; see Table 3.4 for appropriate conversion recommendations.

Comparison of the time-to-maximum serum concentration for OTFC and FBT suggest that FBT should be more rapid in onset than OTFC [74]; however, direct, head-to-head studies of time-to-onset of pain relief have not been done to confirm this. Additionally, FBT has been shown to provide relief of cBTP more rapidly than oxycodone [84].

Fentanyl sublingual tablet

FST is a rapidly dissolving (10–15 seconds) sublingual tablet, containing the active ingredient fentanyl attached to bioadhesive (polyvinylpyrrolidone)-coated carrier particles. The design of FST utilizes an ordered mixture of fine, fentanyl-coated particles that are attached to coarser inactive carrier particles. A bioadhesive is used to increase retention of the fentanyl at the site of absorption (ie, the sublingual mucosa [Figure 3.4]). Once the unit contacts saliva, there is rapid disintegration of the tablet with release of the bioadhesive and fentanyl-carrier particles, which adhere to the sublingual mucosa [85]. The bioadhesive helps to hold the fentanyl in contact with the oral mucosa and prevents the drug from being swallowed, which enhances absorption of the fentanyl [85].

FST has been shown to be effective in the treatment of cBTP [27,86,87]. After a single dose of FST, plasma concentrations of fentanyl have been detected within 10 minutes [85]. Another study evaluating the pharmacokinetics and tolerability of different doses of FST found the first detectable plasma concentration of fentanyl at 8–11 min after FST administration [88]. In one study, improvement in pain control was evident as soon as 5 minutes following administration of FST, although this trend did not become statistically significant until 15 minutes after administration ($P=0.005$) [46]. Another study showed significantly better pain intensity difference scores from 10 minutes after administration of FST compared with placebo ($P=0.0055$); this difference was sustained for 60 minutes [27].

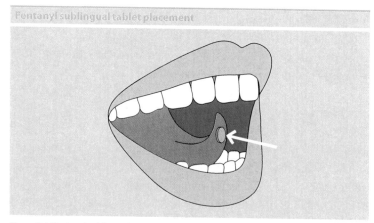

Figure 3.4 Fentanyl sublingual tablet placement. Fentanyl sublingual tablet comes in blister packs and is placed under the tongue for absorption through the sublingual mucosa.

Absorption of fentanyl from FST is mainly through the oral mucosa with a bioavailability calculated to be 54% [8]. In patients who have a dry mouth, water may be used to moisten the buccal mucosa before taking FST. Tablets should be placed on the floor of the mouth directly under the tongue immediately after removal from the blister unit. The tablets should not be chewed, sucked, or swallowed, and should be allowed to completely dissolve in the sublingual cavity. Patients should be advised not to eat or drink anything until the tablet is completely dissolved [8].

While bitter taste is a common complaint among patients using opioids, several studies found that patients taking FST did not have substantial complaints regarding taste [88,89]. There are no masking agents (sugar, flavorings) in FST, although it does contain mannitol, which has a sweet flavor. In one study, 85% of patients indicated that FST was tasteless or virtually tasteless with the majority of other responses indicating a moderately sweet taste [89]. No patients reported gagging associated with FST, and 60% did not detect an aftertaste. Among the 40% of patients who reported an aftertaste, the maximum intensity was mild, with the duration ranging from 1 to 30 minutes [89]. All these patients were willing to continue long-term use of FST [89]. The majority of patients found the drug acceptable from a taste/oral sensation perspective [89]. Another study also confirmed the lack of a bitter taste with FST [88]; however, I have had an occasional patient complain of a bitter, unpleasant taste with FST.

To date there have been no published studies addressing FST use in patients with oral mucositis or xerostomia.

Fentanyl sublingual tablet and titration

FST is supplied in tablets of 100, 200, 300, 400, 600, and 800 µg, and should be titrated upwardly to find the appropriate dose for a patient with cBTP. The 100–400-µg doses come in packs of 12 or 32 tablets. The 600- and 800-µg doses only come in packs of 32 tablets. Similar to the other ROOs, the final titrated dose of FST for cBTP was not predicted from the daily maintenance dose of opioid used to manage the persistent cancer pain. Also, FST shows linear kinetics [88]. For further information on titration of FST, please refer to its package insert [8].

Fentanyl sublingual tablet and other rapid-onset opioids

One of the clinical advantages of FST over OTFC or FBT is that the tablet dissolves quickly, reducing the need for patients to manipulate a lozenge on a stick (OTFC) or to leave a buccal tablet in place for 14–25 minutes (FBT). However, the rapid dissolution of FST means that if there is an immediate, intense opioid effect, then there is no way to terminate delivery of the drug. This is in contrast to OTFC and FBT, where with OTFC the unit can be easily removed from the mouth and with FBT the residual tablet can be scraped and rinsed out of the mouth. Nonetheless, sublingual administration with FST is simpler than the approaches required with OTFC, FBT, or FBSF (where fentanyl is applied through a soluble film, discussed further in the chapter).

Fentanyl pectin nasal spray

FPNS is provided in 5.3-mL clear glass bottles. Each bottle has an attached metered-dose nasal spray pump incorporating a visual- and audible-spray counter, and a protective dust cover. Each bottle contains a net fill weight of 1.57 grams and, after priming, delivers 8 sprays of 100 µL. The pump remains primed for up to 5 days after priming for use. There are 2 product strengths and each 100-µL spray contains either 100 µg or 400 µg of fentanyl. Each bottle is supplied in a child-resistant container. Bottles in their child-resistant containers are supplied in cartons containing 1 or 4 bottles with instructions for use. Each carton contains one carbon-lined pouch per bottle for disposal of priming sprays, unwanted doses, and residual fentanyl solution. Like FSS, FPNS comes in a rather bulky childproof container and transportation of more than a few days' supply of medication might pose some difficulties for patients.

FPNS uses a pectin-based gelling agent (PecSys® delivery system) to provide a controlled release of fentanyl across the nasal mucosa through a spray; this drug-delivery system enhances the transmucosal fentanyl absorption and produces a consistent fentanyl-plasma concentration (Figure 3.5) [22,90]. The pectin-based gelling system allows the aqueous

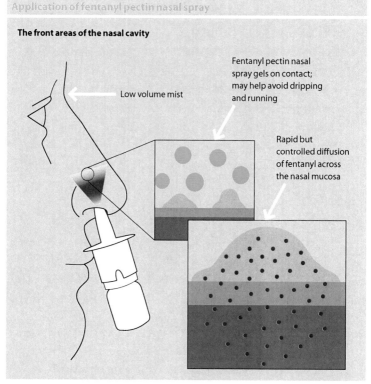

Figure 3.5 Application of fentanyl pectin nasal spray. Fentanyl pectin nasal spray uses a pectin-based gelling system to control absorption via the nasal mucosa.

solution (ie, carboxylic acid) in the spray bottle to turn into a gel when sprayed onto mucosal surfaces (ie, when the spray comes in contact with calcium ions in the nasal mucosa). The fentanyl is held in this gel matrix and released by simple diffusion onto the nasal mucosa. The diffusion from the gel controls the deposition of fentanyl onto the nasal mucosa and the gel also prevents the fentanyl from "running off" into the posterior pharynx to be swallowed. The natural action of the nasal cilia does eventually move the gel to the posterior pharynx where it is swallowed. The process of fentanyl diffusion from the gel matrix is thought to blunt the peak plasma level of fentanyl when compared to a simple aqueous-based fentanyl nasal spray. This may help prevent adverse events associated with high peak plasma levels of drug.

With administration of a nasal drug, one might be concerned about alteration of absorption with allergic rhinitis. Studies have shown that fentanyl absorption is not affected by the presence of allergic rhinitis; however, coadministration of a vasoconstricting nasal decongestant leads to lower peak fentanyl plasma concentrations and a delayed time to maximum concentration that may cause FPNS to be less effective. Additionally, titration of a patient while they are using a vasoconstricting decongestant might lead to incorrect dosing such that once the vasoconstrictor is stopped drug absorption might improve and the patient may receive too large of a dose [12,13].

Fentanyl pectin nasal spray and titration

FPNS dose titration is performed in a manner similar to other ROOs. As with the sublingual and buccal ROOs, linear pharmacokinetics apply [91]. The initial dose is 100 µg delivered as one spray in one nostril. The second step in titration is 200 µg delivered as one 100-µg spray in each nostril. The next dose is 400 µg delivered as one spray in one nostril. This is followed by 800 µg delivered as one spray of the 400-µg dose in each nostril. The safety and efficacy of doses higher than 800 µg have not been evaluated in clinical studies. There are no clinical data to support the use of a combination of dose strengths to treat cBTP episodes [91]. For more information regarding titration for FPNS, please refer to package inserts [12,13].

A study that examined the effects of dosing intervals shorter than the recommended 4 hours showed that there was a stacking effect. In other words, a higher maximum serum concentration occurred if a second dose was administered 1 or 2 hours after the initial dose. This increase in maximum concentration was not seen with a 4-hour interval between doses. This study suggests a minimum of a 2-hour interval between FPNS doses. This same study looked at the effects of delivering 8 sprays into one nostril. The blood levels were not dose proportional in this latter situation, suggesting that the capacity of the nasal cavity might have been exceeded and that unabsorbed fentanyl may have run off into the pharynx and had been swallowed [22]. It is not known if this confers a safety benefit to this mode of fentanyl delivery.

Fentanyl pectin nasal spray and other rapid-onset opioids

Many patients with cancer may not tolerate oral medications. FPNS may be particularly useful when the patient is at risk of oral mucositis, dry mouth, and/or nausea with oral medications. Patients who receive radiation treatment for head and neck cancer often suffer from dry mouth due to the effects of radiation on the parotid and salivary glands; nausea is very common in patients with cancer and sometimes oral medications exacerbate these events. Given the general efficacy, safety, and acceptability of FPNS for the management of cBTP episodes [47,92–94], the nasal approach of FPNS may be beneficial for this group of patients [95].

Fentanyl pectin nasal spray and comparative clinical trials

In a head-to-head study with oral morphine, FPNS provided more rapid onset of analgesia (30 minutes [$P<0.01$] and 60 minutes [$P<0.05$]) and had higher acceptability scores than oral morphine [96]. There were no significant nasal effects from the drug in this study [96]. In long-term studies to assess nasal and general tolerability, FPNS was generally well-tolerated and there was no evidence of nasal toxicity [93,97]. In a study comparing FPNS to oral morphine, FPNS significantly improved the mean pain intensity difference score at 15 minutes and 57.5% of FPNS-treated cBTP episodes demonstrated onset of pain relief by 5 minutes and 95.7% by 30 minutes [98]. The cBTP intensity decreased by 2 or more points by 10 minutes in 52.4% of patients treated; no significant nasal effects were reported [98]. In a study comparing FPNS to placebo, 33% of FPNS treated cBTP episodes showed an onset of improvement in pain intensity at 5 minutes, and by 10 minutes 33% of episodes had clinically meaningful pain relief. At the end of the study, 87% of patients elected to continue treatment with FPNS, reflecting the fact that FPNS was well-accepted by the patients [47,92]. A long-term safety study included nasal assessments, which did not reveal any clinically significant effects on the nasal mucosa [93].

Fentanyl pectin nasal spray and oral transmucosal fentanyl citrate
Fentanyl administered as FPNS is more rapidly absorbed, reaches higher maximum plasma concentrations, and has an approximately 20% greater bioavailability than OTFC [12,13,99]. In a preclinical trial to assess different gelling agents, the pectin-based intranasal delivery system demonstrated significantly increased systemic fentanyl exposure and reduced times to peak fentanyl plasma values compared with OTFC [100].

Fentanyl buccal soluble film
FBSF uses the BioErodible MucoAdhesive (BEMA™) [101] bilayer-delivery technology to transport fentanyl across the buccal mucosa. Each film is individually wrapped in a child-resistant, protective foil package. These foil packages are packed 30 per carton. The BEMA technology is based on multilayer water-soluble polymeric films, comprised of bioerodible polymers. FBSF consists of a pink bioadhesive layer (mucosal side), which is bonded onto a white inactive layer (oral-cavity side) (Figure 3.6) [101]. The fentanyl is incorporated into the bioadhesive layer, which readily adheres to the buccal mucosa upon contact, the film further softens with moisture, rapidly becoming unnoticeable. Once applied, the BEMA disc immediately begins to deliver fentanyl. The backing layer of the film, facing outward toward the oral cavity, minimizes drug release into the oral cavity because of its occlusive properties, thereby maximizing delivery of fentanyl into the mucosal tissue [102–104]. Once the backing layer fully erodes (typically in less than 30 minutes after application),

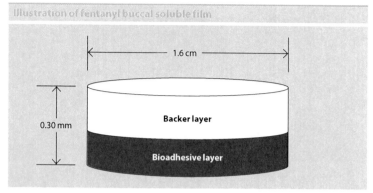

Figure 3.6 Illustration of fentanyl buccal soluble film. In fentanyl buccal soluble film, through BioErodible MucoAdhesive technology, fentanyl is incorporated into the bioadhesive layer, which is applied to the buccal mucosa. Adapted from Cox [101].

the bioadhesive layer, adherent to the mucosa, dissolves quickly, leaving no residue at the application site [104].

Prior to administration of the film, the patient should use the tongue or rinse the mouth with water to wet the area for placement of FSBF (Figure 3.7). The patient should be instructed to place the pink, bioadhesive side of the FBSF against the inside of the cheek, and press and hold the film in place for 5 seconds; the film should stay in place on its own after this period. Liquids may be consumed after 5 minutes. The FBSF will dissolve within 15–30 minutes after application. The film should not be manipulated with the tongue or finger(s), and eating food should be avoided until the film has dissolved [104].

FBSF has an absolute bioavailability of 71% with 51% of a dose absorbed through the buccal mucosa [104]. The amount of fentanyl delivered transmucosally is proportional to the film surface area, thus larger doses require larger patches [14]. This direct relationship (between surface area and the dose) results in consistent plasma concentrations when equivalent doses are delivered by single or multiple dosage units; like other ROOs, the pharmacokinetics of FBSF are linear [104,105]. This is illustrated by the fact that the buccal surface area covered by a single 800-μg dose is the same surface area covered by four individual 200-μg films [104].

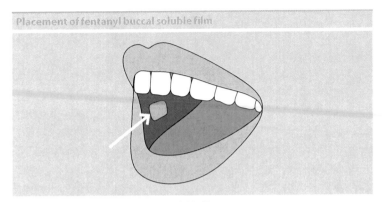

Figure 3.7 Placement of fentanyl buccal soluble film.

In clinical trials FBSF has been shown to be effective for the treatment of cBTP [14]. It was well-tolerated in the oral cavity, with no treatment-related oral adverse effects [48]. Furthermore, FBSF was evaluated in a group of patients (n=7) with grade 1 oral mucositis and a matched group of control patients (n=7) without oral mucositis. The adverse event profile was similar in both groups of patients. There was no evidence that FBSF caused or worsened oral-mucosal irritation or pain in either study group. The maximum concentration of drug was slightly less in the mucositis group [106]. However, it must be noted that this was only mild, grade 1 mucositis and caution should be used if selecting this drug for patients with more severe oral mucositis.

Fentanyl buccal soluble film and titration

FBSF is available in doses of 200, 400, 600, 800, and 1200 µg. It is recommended that FBSF be titrated upward from the lowest dose to find the appropriate dose for the patient. Please see package insert for specific titration instructions for FBSF [14].

Fentanyl buccal soluble film and other rapid-onset opioids

Compared to OTFC, FBSF produces faster and more efficient transmucosal fentanyl delivery, yielding a shorter time to maximum concentration, higher maximum concentration (62% greater maximum plasma concentration), and greater bioavailability [103].

Fentanyl sublingual spray

FSS is a single-dose device that delivers a 100-µL spray for the sublingual administration of fentanyl. FSS is applied to the thin, highly vascular sublingual mucosa for delivery of nonionic fentanyl [21].The sublingual mucosa is more permeable than the buccal mucosa because of differences in thickness between the sublingual and the buccal mucosal membranes, the sublingual mucous membrane being significantly thinner than the buccal membrane [107]. FSS has a bioavailability of 76% [15]. Each 100-µL spray produces a fine mist that covers the sublingual mucosa (Figure 3.8). The patient should be instructed to squeeze the spray between their finger and thumb, directing the spray under their tongue. The medicine should be held under their tongue for 30–60 second during which time they should not spit out or rinse their mouths [29].

FSS might not be the ideal drug for patients with oral mucositis. The package insert for FSS reports increases in fentanyl absorption in patients with grade 1 and grade 2 oral mucositis [15]. Patients with grade 2 mucositis had a 4–7 times higher maximum concentration than those without mucositis [15]. Thus, there is the risk of unintentional overdose

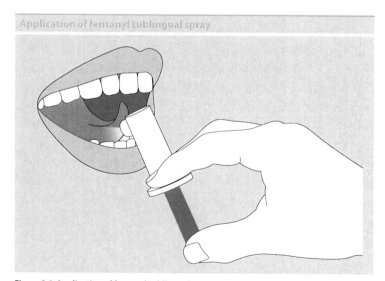

Application of fentanyl sublingual spray

Figure 3.8 Application of fentanyl sublingual spray. In patients with normal dentation, the nozzle of the applicator may be seated against the lower teeth to assist the patient with directing the spray onto the sublingual mucosa.

if FSS is used in patients with mucositis [15]. The smell of ethanol may be detectable with the activation of the FSS unit and theoretically this smell might trigger alcohol cravings in patients with alcoholism.

Fentanyl sublingual spray and titration
Like other ROOs, the FSS should be titrated upward from the lowest dose until an appropriate dose is found to manage the cBTP episodes for the patient. FSS is provided in dose packs of 100, 200, 400, 600, 800, 1200, and 1600 μg; different doses have different colored activators and plungers. The 1200- and 1600-μg doses are supplied as two 600- or two 800-μg doses, respectively, in one childproof blister package. The 1200- and 1600-μg doses are produced by sequential administration of the 600- or 800-μg doses. Each dose is color coded and the 1200- and 1600-μg "dual unit" doses are color coded differently than the individual 600- and 800-μg doses. Please see package insert for specific titration instructions for FSS [15].

Fentanyl sublingual spray and comparative clinical trials
In a randomized, double-blind placebo-controlled Phase III trial, FSS produced a significant reduction in pain intensity within 5 minutes of administration that persisted through the 60-minute study period ($P<0.0001$) [21]. To date, this drug may produce the most rapid onset of analgesic effect of all the transmucosal fentanyl medications. During the open-label titration period, 75.4% of patients found a successful dose. At the end of the study, 94.7% of patients choose to continue in a long-term safety study, reflecting their satisfaction with FSS compared to their previous cBTP medications. Also, most patients found the sublingual spray convenient and easy to use [21]. Another study in patients with cBTP also reported that better analgesia was achieved with FSS compared to placebo; the study reported the median dose of fentanyl as 800 μg (range: 100–1600 μg) [108].

FSS may be particularly advantageous for certain patients with cancer who might benefit from the 5-minute onset of analgesia. For example, a patient who is awoken at night in severe pain at the peak of a cBTP episode might benefit more from the rapid onset of analgesia from FSS compared to the other cBTP medications. Additionally, as dry mouth is common in patients with cancer, FSS should offer an advantage over the ROOs that require moisture for dissolution.

Intranasal fentanyl spray

Intranasal fentanyl spray (INFS) was approved throughout the European Union in 2011. It is not yet approved in the United States. INFS is applied by the patient inserting the spray nozzle into one nostril while holding down the other. The spray coats the transmucosal lining of the nasal cavity, and should take effect after approximately 5–6 minutes; the bioavailability of INFS is 89% [11]. Along with FSS and FPNS, INFS represents one of the shortest onset times possible with transmucosal drugs. Given that the entry time for fentanyl into the central nervous system across the blood–brain barrier is thought to be about 5 or 6 minutes [17], it is unlikely that transmucosal drugs will provide much faster onset of action than is seen with these two fentanyl formulations. Pulmonary delivery of fentanyl may produce faster onset-of-action, identical to intravenous delivery, but such systems are not yet clinically available and it is not likely that a pulmonary fentanyl or similar product will be available in the near future [107,108].

In clinical trials with INFS there was one report of nasal ulceration, which rapidly healed following cessation of therapy [109] and one report of a nose bleed [50].

Intranasal fentanyl spray and titration

INFS should be titrated upward from the lowest dose to find the appropriate pain relief for patients with cBTP; please see the package insert for specific titration instructions [11]. INFS is supplied in 50-, 100-, and 200-µg doses in packs of 2, 6, 8, and 10 containers. INFS also comes in the same strengths in multidose vials, containing 10 or 20 doses per vial [11].

Intranasal fentanyl spray and oral transmucosal fentanyl citrate

In one study of cBTP episodes treated with INFS, the median time to onset of "meaningful" pain relief was 11 minutes with INFS versus 16 minutes with OTFC, and 65.7% of patients attained faster time to "meaningful" pain-relief onset with INFS compared to OTFC [109]. This study also found that significantly more patients achieved meaningful pain relief at 5 minutes with INFS: 25.3% for INFS versus 6.8% for OTFC ($P<0.001$) [109]. It appears that INFS provides a faster onset of analgesic action than OTFC.

Summary

The development of the ROOs has marked a new era in cancer pain management. Prior to the introduction of the first ROO, there were no oral medications that were able to satisfactorily address spontaneous cBTP episodes with rapid onset of intense pain. As Perry Fine pointed out in 1995 when discussing early clinical trials of OTFC for cBTP, "if this dosage form proves to be effective in this population, a major hurdle in the palliation of cancer pain will have been overcome" [110]. The ability for patients to use highly effective oral analgesics that can work as rapidly as intravenous morphine is a miracle of modern pharmacology and a tremendous benefit to patients with cancer suffering with cBTP. Optimal use of these medications requires that one understand the unique pharmacological profiles associated with the different formulations. Application of simple-dosing guidelines, good communication with the patient and caregiver, and utilization of the well-established principles of "for the individual" and with "attention to detail" allows the practitioner to use these drugs for the benefit of patients suffering from cBTP.

References

1   Actiq [package insert]. Frazer, PA: Cephalon, Inc; 2011.
2   Vallejo R, Barkin RL, Wang, VC. Pharmacology of opioids in the treatment of chronic pain syndromes. *Pain Physician*. 2011;14:E343-E360.
3   Stanley TH. The history and development of the fentanyl series. *J Pain Symptom Manage*. 1992;7(3 Suppl):S3-S7.
4   Roy SD, Flynn GL. Transdermal delivery of narcotic analgesics: pH, anatomical, and subject influences on cutaneous permeability of fentanyl and sufentanil. *Pharm Res*. 1990;7:842-847.
5   Grond S, Radbruch L, Lehmann KA. Clinical pharmacokinetics of transdermal opioids: focus on transdermal fentanyl. *Clin Pharmacokinet*. 2000;38:59-89.
6   Stanley TH. Fentanyl. *J Pain Symptom Manage*. 2005;29:S67-S71.
7   Mystakidou K, Tsilika E, Tsiatas M, Vlahos L. Oral transmucosal fentanyl citrate in cancer pain management: a practical application of nanotechnology. *Int J Nanomedicine*. 2007;2:49-54.

8   Abstral [package insert]. Bridgewater, NJ: ProStrakan Inc.; 2012.

9   Fentora [package insert]. Frazer, PA: Cephalon, Inc.; 2011.

10 Effentora [package insert]. Maisons-Alfort, France: Cephalon France; 2012.

11 Instanyl [package insert]. Roskilde, Denmark: Nycomed Danmark ApS; 2012.

12 Lazanda [package insert]. Bedminster, NJ: Archimedes Pharma US Inc.; 2012.

13 PecFent [package insert]. Scandicci, Italy: Archimedes Development Ltd; 2012.

14 Onsolis [package insert]. Franklin Township, NJ: Meda Pharmaceuticals; 2012.

15 Subsys [package insert]. Phoenix, AZ: INSYS Therapeutics, Inc.; 2012.

16 Streisand JB, Varvel JR, Stanski DR, et al. Absorption and bioavailability of oral transmucosal fentanyl citrate. *Anesthesiology*. 1991;75:223-229.

17 Scott JC, Ponganis KV, Stanski DR. EEG quantification of narcotic effect: The comparative pharmacodynamics of fentanyl and alfentanil. *Anesthesiology*. 1985;62:234-241.

18 Csaba N, Garcia-Fuentes M, Alonso MJ. The performance of nanocarriers for transmucosal drug delivery. *Expert Opin Drug Deliv*. 2006;3:463-478.

19 Durfee S, Messina J, Khankari R. Fentanyl effervescent buccal tablets: enhanced buccal absorption. *Am J Drug Deliv*. 2006;4:1-5.

20 Darwish M, Kirby M, Robertson P Jr, Tracewell W, Jiang JG. Absolute and relative bioavailability of fentanyl buccal tablet and oral transmucosal fentanyl citrate. *J Clin Pharmacol*. 2007;47:343-350.

21 Rauck R, Reynolds L, Bull J, et al. Efficacy and safety of fentanyl sublingual spray for the treatment of breakthrough cancer pain: a randomized, double-blind, placebo-controlled study. *Curr Med Res Opin*. 2012;28:859-870.

22 Taylor D, Gabrail N. Fentanyl pectin nasal spray for breakthrough cancer pain. *Future Oncol*. 2012;8:121-130.

23 Zeppetella G. Breakthrough Pain in Cancer Patients. *Clin Oncol*. 23:393-398.

24 Christie JM, Simmonds M, Patt R, Coluzzi P, et al. Dose-titration, multicenter study of oral transmucosal fentanyl citrate for the treatment of breakthrough pain in cancer patients using transdermal fentanyl for persistent pain. *J Clin Oncol*. 1998;16:3238-3245.

25 Messina J, Darwish M, Fine PG. Fentanyl buccal tablet. *Drugs Today (Barc)*. 2008;44:41-54.

26 Zeppetella G. Opioids for cancer breakthrough pain: a pilot study reporting patient assessment of time to meaningful pain relief. *J Pain Symptom Manage*. 2008;35:563-567.

27 Rauck RL, Tark M, Reyes E, et al. Efficacy and long-term tolerability of sublingual fentanyl orally disintegrating tablet in the treatment of breakthrough cancer pain. *Curr Med Res Opin*. 2009;25:2877-2885.

28 Mercadante S, Ferrera P, Adile C, Casuccio A. Fentanyl buccal tablets for breakthrough pain in highly tolerant cancer patients: preliminary data on the proportionality between breakthrough pain dose and background dose. *J Pain Symptom Manage*. 2011;42:464-469.

29 Mercadante S. The use of rapid onset opioids for breakthrough cancer pain: The challenge of its dosing. *Crit Rev Oncol Hematol*. 2011;80:460-465.

30 Davies AN, Dickman A, Reid C, Stevens AM, Zeppetella G; Science Committee of the Association for Palliative Medicine of Great Britain and Ireland. The management of cancer-related breakthrough pain: recommendations of a task group of the Science Committee of the Association for Palliative Medicine of Great Britain and Ireland. *Eur J Pain*. 2009;13:331-338.

31 Farrar JT Cleary J, Rauck R. Oral transmucosal fentanyl citrate: randomized, double-blinded, placebo-controlled trial for treatment of breakthrough pain in cancer patients. *J Natl Cancer Inst*. 1998;90:611-616.

32 Hagen NA, Fisher K, Victorino C, Farrar JT. A titration strategy is needed to manage breakthrough cancer pain effectively: observations from data pooled from three clinical trials. *J Palliat Med*. 2007;10:47-55.

33 Jost L, Roila F; ESMO Guidelines Working Group. Management of cancer pain: ESMO clinical recommendations. *Ann Oncol*. 2008;19 Suppl 2:ii119-121.

34 Mercadante S, Villari P, Ferrera P, Casuccio A. Optimization of opioid therapy for preventing incident pain associated with bone metastases. *J Pain Symptom Manage.* 2004;28:505-510.

35 Payne R, Coluzzi P, Hart L, et al. Long-term safety of oral transmucosal fentanyl citrate for breakthrough cancer pain. *J Pain Symptom Manage.* 2001;22:575-583.

36 Chaushu G, Bercovici M, Dori S, et al. Salivary flow and its relation with oral symptoms in terminally ill patients. *Cancer.* 2000;88:984-987.

37 Elting LS, Keefe DM, Sonis ST, et al; Burden of Illness Head and Neck Writing Committee. Patient-reported measurements of oral mucositis in head and neck cancer patients treated with radiotherapy with or without chemotherapy: demonstration of increased frequency, severity, resistance to palliation, and impact on quality of life. *Cancer.* 2008;113:2704-2713.

38 Caraceni A, Zecca E, Bonezzi C, et al. Gabapentin for neuropathic cancer pain: a randomized controlled trial from the Gabapentin Cancer Pain Study Group. *J Clin Oncol.* 2004;22:2909-2917.

39 National Cancer Institute. Pain (PDQ®) Health Professional Version. www.cancer.gov/cancertopics/pdq/supportivecare/pain/HealthProfessional/page1. Accessed February 1, 2013.

40 Bennett D, Burton AW, Fishman S, et al. Consensus panel recommendations for the assessment and management of breakthrough pain: Part 2 Management. *P T.* 2005;30:354-361.

41 Chrvala CA, Caspi A. P&T product profiler Abstral® (fentanyl sublingual tablets for breakthrough cancer pain). *P T.* 2011;36:1-28.

42 Pergolizzi J, Raffa RB. Common opioid-drug interactions: what clinicians need to know. In: Tollison CD, Satterthwaite Jr, Tollison JW, eds. *Practical Pain Management.* Philadelphia, PA: Lippincott Williams and Wilkins; 2011:1-54.

43 Ashburn MA, Lind GH, Gillie MH, de Boer AJ, Pace NL, Stanley TH. Oral transmucosal fentanyl citrate (OTFC) for the treatment of postoperative pain. *Anesth Analg.* 1993;76:377-381.

44 Mercadante S. Managing Breakthrough Pain. *Curr Pain Headache Rep.* 2011;15:244-249.

45 Portenoy R, Taylor D, Messina J, Tremmel L. A randomized, placebo-controlled study of fentanyl buccal tablet for breakthrough pain in opioid-treated patients with cancer. *Clin J Pain.* 2006;22:805-811.

46 Lennernäs B, Frank-Lissbrant I, Lennernäs H, Kälkner KM, Derrick R, Howell J. Sublingual administration of fentanyl to cancer patients is an effective treatment for breakthrough pain: results from a randomized phase II study. *Palliat Med.* 2010;24:286-293.

47 Taylor D, Galan V, Weinstein SM, Reyes E, Pupo-Araya AR, Rauck R; Fentanyl Pectin Nasal Spray 043 Study Group. Fentanyl pectin nasal spray in breakthrough cancer pain. *J Support Oncol.* 2010;8:184-190.

48 Rauck R, North J, Gever LN, Tagarro I, Finn AL. Fentanyl buccal soluble film (FBSF) for breakthrough pain in patients with cancer: a randomized, double-blind, placebo-controlled study. *Ann Oncol.* 2010;21:1308-1314.

49 Nalamachu S, Hassman D, Wallace MS, Dumble S, Derrick R, Howell J. Long-term effectiveness and tolerability of sublingual fentanyl orally disintegrating tablet for the treatment of breakthrough cancer pain. *Curr Med Res Opin.* 2011;27:519-530.

50 Kress HG, Ororiska A, Kaczmarek Z, Kaasa S, Colberg T, Nolte T. Efficacy and tolerability of intranasal fentanyl spray 50 to 200 microg for breakthrough pain in patients with cancer: a phase III, multinational, randomized, double-blind, placebo-controlled, crossover trial with a la-month, open-label extension treatment period. *Clin Ther.* 2009;31:1177-1191.

51 Landy SH. Oral transmucosal fentanyl citrate for the treatment of migraine headache pain in outpatients: a case series. *Headache.* 2004;44:762-766.

52 Lind GH, Marcus MA, Mears SL, et al. Oral transmucosal fentanyl citrate for analgesia and sedation in the emergency department. *Ann Emerg Med.* 1991;20:1117-1120.

53 Davies AN, Vriens J, Kennett A, McTaggart M. An observational study of oncology patients' utilization of breakthrough pain medication. *J Pain Symptom Manage.* 2008;35:406-411.

54 Shaiova L, Lapin J, Manco LS, et al. Tolerability and effects of two formulations of oral transmucosal fentanyl citrate (OTFC; ACTIQ) in patients with radiation-induced oral mucositis. *Support Care Cancer*. 2004;12:268-273.

55 Ashburn MA, Fine PG, Stanley TH. Oral transmucosal fentanyl citrate for the treatment of breakthrough cancer pain: a case report. *Anesthesiology*. 1989;71:615-617.

56 Medication Guide. Oral Transmucosal Fentanyl Citrate (OTFC) CII (fentanyl citrate) oral transmucosal lozenge 200 mcg, 400 mcg, 600 mcg, 800 mcg, 1200 mcg, 1600 mcg. www.tirfremsaccess.com/TirfUI/rems/pdf/anesta-medication-guide.pdf. Updated December 2011. Accessed February 1, 2013.

57 Gee SS, Cunningham J, Rome J, Reid K. Dental disease and the use of oral transmucosal fentanyl: a case report. Presented at: American Academy of Pain Medicine 23rd Annual Meeting; February 7–10, 2007; New Orleans, LA.

58 Mandel L, Carunchio MJ. Rampant caries from oral transmucosal fentanyl citrate lozenge abuse. *J Am Dent Assoc*. 2011;142:406-409.

59 Mystakidou K, Katsouda E, Parpa E, Vlahos L, Tsiatas ML. Oral transmucosal fentanyl citrate: overview of pharmacological and clinical characteristics. *Drug Deliv*. 2006;13:269-276.

60 Mystakidou K, Katsouda E, Parpa E, Tsiatas ML, Vlahos L. Oral transmucosal fentanyl citrate for the treatment of breakthrough pain in cancer patients: an overview of its pharmacological and clinical characteristics. *Am J Hosp Palliat Care*. 2005;22:228-232.

61 McMenamin E, Farrar JT. Oral transmucosal fentanyl citrate: a novel agent for breakthrough pain related to cancer. *Expert Rev Neurother*. 2002;2:625-629.

62 Portenoy RK, Payne R, Coluzzi P, et al. Oral transmucosal fentanyl citrate (OTFC) for the treatment of breakthrough pain in cancer patients: a controlled dose titration study. *Pain*. 1999;79:303-312.

63 Mercadante S, Villari P, Ferrera P, Mangione S, Casuccio A. The use of opioids for breakthrough pain in acute palliative care unit by using doses proportional to opioid basal regimen. *Clin J Pain*. 2010;26:306-309.

64 Coluzzi P, Schwartzberg L, Conroy J, et al. Breakthrough cancer pain: a randomized trial comparing oral transmucosal fentanyl citrate (OTFC) and morphine sulfate immediate release (MSIR). *Pain*. 2001;91:123-130.

65 Streisand JB, Busch MA, Egan TD, Smith BG, Gay M, Pace NL. Dose proportionality and pharmacokinetics of oral transmucosal fentanyl citrate. *Anesthesiology*. 1998;88:305-309.

66 Aronoff G, Brennan M, Pritchard D, Ginsberg B. Evidence based oral transmucosal fentanyl citrate (OTFC) dosing guidelines. *Pain Med*. 2005;6:305-314.

67 Lichtor JL, Sevarino, FB, Joshi GP, Busch MA, Nordbrock E, Ginsberg B. The relative potency of oral transmucosal fentanyl citrate compared with intravenous morphine in the treatment of moderate to severe postoperative pain. *Anesth Analg*. 1999;89:732-738.

68 Kotwal RS, O'Connor KC, Johnson TR, Mosely DS, Meyer DE, Holcomb JB. Novel pain management strategy for combat casualty care. *Ann Emerg Med*. 2004;44:121-127.

69 Darwish M, Xie F. Pharmacokinetics of fentanyl buccal tablet: a pooled analysis and review. *Pain Pract*. 2012;12:307-314.

70 Darwish M, Kirby M, Jiang JG, Tracewell W, Robertson P Jr. Bioequivalence following buccal and sublingual placement of fentanyl buccal tablet 400 microg in healthy subjects. *Clin Drug Investig*. 2008;28:1-7.

71 Pather I, Siebert JM, Hontz J, Khankari R, Gupte S. Enhanced buccal delivery of fentanyl using the oravescent drug delivery system. Drug Development & Delivery. www.drugdeliverytech.com/ME2/dirmod.asp?sid=&nm=&type=Publishing&mod=Publica tions%3A%3AArticle&mid=8F3A7027421841978F18BE895F87F791&tier=4&id=59F509813 D564E318080426DC9513DD7. Published October 2001. Accessed February 1, 2013.

72 Breakthrough Cancer Pain. www.breakthroughcancerpain.org. Accessed February 1, 2013.

73 Darwish M, Kirby M, Jiang JG. Effect of buccal dwell time on the pharmacokinetic profile of fentanyl buccal tablet. *Expert Opin Pharmacother*. 2007;8:2011-2016.

74   Freye E. A new transmucosal drug delivery system for patients with breakthrough cancer pain: the fentanyl effervescent buccal tablet. *J Pain Res*. 2008;2:13-20.

75   Medication Guide. FENTORA® (fen-tor-a) CII (fentanyl citrate) buccal tablet 100 mcg, 200 mcg, 400 mcg, 600 mcg, 800 mcg. www.fda.gov/downloads/Drugs/DrugSafety/ucm088597.pdf. Published December 2011. Accessed February 1, 2013.

76   Darwish M, Kirby M, Robertson P Jr, Tracewell W, Xie F. Dose proportionality of fentanyl buccal tablet in doses ranging from 600 to 1300 microg in healthy adult subjects: a randomized, open-label, four-period, crossover, single-centre study. *Clin Drug Investig*. 2010;30:365-373.

77   Darwish M, Tempero K, Kirby M, Thompson J. Relative bioavailability of the fentanyl effervescent buccal tablet (FEBT) 1,080 pg versus oral transmucosal fentanyl citrate 1,600 pg and dose proportionality of FEBT 270 to 1,300 microg: a single-dose, randomized, open-label, three-period study in healthy adult volunteers. *Clin Ther*. 2006;28:715-724.

78   Darwish M, Kirby M, Robertson P, Tracewell W, Jiang JG. Absorption of fentanyl from fentanyl buccal tablet in cancer patients with or without oral mucositis: a pilot study. *Clin Drug Investig*. 2007;27:605-611.

79   Weinstein SM, Messina J, Xie F. Fentanyl buccal tablet for the treatment of breakthrough pain in opioid-tolerant patients with chronic cancer pain: A long-term, open-label safety study. *Cancer*. 2009;115:2571-2579.

80   Mercadante S, Ferrera P, Arcuri E. The use of fentanyl buccal tablets as breakthrough medication in patients receiving chronic methadone therapy: an open label preliminary study. *Support Care Cancer*. 2011;19:435-438.

81   Zeppetella G, Messina J, Xie F, Slatkin NE. Consistent and clinically relevant effects with fentanyl buccal tablet in the treatment of patients receiving maintenance opioid therapy and experiencing cancer-related breakthrough pain. *Pain Pract*. 2010;10:287-293.

82   Slatkin NE, Xie F, Messina J, Segal TJ. Fentanyl buccal tablet for relief of breakthrough pain in opioid-tolerant patients with cancer-related chronic pain. *J Support Oncol*. 2007;5:327-334.

83   Lecybyl R, Hanna M. Fentanyl buccal tablet: faster rescue analgesia for breakthrough pain? *Future Oncol*. 2007;3:375-379.

84   Ashburn MA, Slevin KA, Messina J, Xie F. The efficacy and safety of fentanyl buccal tablet compared with immediate-release oxycodone for the management of breakthrough pain in opioid-tolerant patients with chronic pain. *Anesth Analg*. 2011;112:693-702.

85   Bredenberg S, Duberg M, Lennernäs B, et al. In vitro and in vivo evaluation of a new sublingual tablet system for rapid oromucosal absorption using fentanyl citrate as the active substance. *Eur J Pharm Sci*. 2003;20:327-334.

86   Nalamachu SR, Rauck RL, Wallace MS, Hassman D, Howell J. Successful dose finding with sublingual fentanyl tablet: combined results from 2 open-label titration studies. *Pain Pract*. 2012;12:449-456.

87   Überall MA, Müller-Schwefe GH. Sublingual fentanyl orally disintegrating tablet in daily practice: efficacy, safety and tolerability in patients with breakthrough cancer pain. *Curr Med Res Opin*. 2011;27:1385-1394.

88   Lennernäs B, Hedner T, Holmberg M, Bredenberg S, Nyström C, Lennernäs H. Pharmacokinetics and tolerability of different doses of fentanyl following sublingual administration of a rapidly dissolving tablet to cancer patients: a new approach to treatment of incident pain. *Br J Clin Pharmacol*. 2005;59:249-253.

89   Lennernäs B, James L, Duberg M, Howell J. Patient acceptability of fentanyl sublingual tablet for the treatment of breakthrough pain. Presented at: American Academy of Pain Management; September 21–24, 2010; Las Vegas, NV.

90   Watts P, Smith A. PecSys: in situ gelling system for optimised nasal drug delivery. *Expert Opin Drug Deliv*. 2009;6:543-552.

91   Fisher T, Watling M, Smith A, Knight A. Pharmacokinetics and relative bioavailability of fentanyl pectin nasal spray 100–800 µg in healthy volunteers. *Int J Clin Pharmacol Ther*. 2010;48:860-867.

92   Portenoy RK, Burton AW, Gabrail N, Taylor D; Fentanyl Pectin Nasal Spray 043 Study Group. A multicenter, placebo-controlled, double-blind, multiple-crossover study of Fentanyl Pectin Nasal Spray (FPNS) in the treatment of breakthrough cancer pain. *Pain*. 2010;151:617-24.

93   Radbruch L, Torres LM, Ellershaw JE, et al. Long-term tolerability, efficacy and acceptability of fentanyl pectin nasal spray for breakthrough cancer pain. *Support Care Cancer*. 2012;20:565-573.

94   Davis G, Knight AC, Love R, Fisher AN. Nasalfent, a novel intranasal formulation of fentanyl, is rapidly effective and well-tolerated during treatment of breakthrough cancer pain. Presented at: 10th Congress of the European Association of Palliative Care; June 7–9, 2007; Budapest, Hungary.

95   Mystakidou K, Panagiotou I, Gouliamos A. Fentanyl nasal spray for the treatment of cancer pain. *Expert Opin Pharmacother*. 2011;12:1653-1659.

96   Davies A, Sitte T, Elsner F, Reale C, Espinosa J, Brooks D, Fallon M. Consistency of efficacy, patient acceptability, and nasal tolerability of fentanyl pectin nasal spray compared with immediate-release morphine sulfate in breakthrough cancer pain. *J Pain Symptom Manage*. 2011;41:358-366.

97   Portenoy RK, Raffaeli W, Torres LM, et al; Fentanyl Nasal Spray Study 045 Investigators Group. Long-term safety, tolerability, and consistency of effect of fentanyl pectin nasal spray for breakthrough cancer pain in opioid-tolerant patients. *J Opioid Manag*. 2010;6:319-328.

98   Fallon M, Reale C, Davies A, et al; Fentanyl Nasal Spray Study 044 Investigators Group. Efficacy and safety of fentanyl pectin nasal spray compared with immediate-release morphine sulfate tablets in the treatment of breakthrough cancer pain: a multicenter, randomized, controlled, double-blind, double-dummy multiple-crossover study. *J Support Oncol*. 2011;9:224-231.

99   Lyseng-Williamson KA. Fentanyl pectin nasal spray: in breakthrough pain in opioid-tolerant adults with cancer. *CNS Drugs*. 2011;25:511-522.

100   Fisher A, Watling M, Smith A, Knight A. Pharmacokinetic comparisons of three nasal fentanyl formulations; pectin, chitosan and chitosan-poloxamer 188. *Int J Clin Pharmacol Ther*. 2010;48:138-145.

101   Cox C. Treatment options gel with innovative drug delivery systems. Drug Development & Delivery. www.drugdeliverytech.com/ME2/dirmod.asp?sid=4306B1E9C3CC4E07A4D64E23 FBDB232C&nm=Back+Issues&type=Publishing&mod=Publications%3A%3AArticle&mid=8 F3A7027421841978F18BE895F87F791&tier=4&id=A1DD814A0D3A443D968BC8B2B4DAA 01D. Published June 2002. Accessed February 1, 2013.

102   Vasisht N, Gever LN, Tagarro I, Finn AL. Evaluation of the single- and multiple-dose pharmacokinetics of fentanyl buccal soluble film in normal healthy volunteers. *J Clin Pharmacol*. 2010;50:785-791.

103   Vasisht N, Gever LN, Tagarro I, Finn AL. Formulation selection and pharmacokinetic comparison of fentanyl buccal soluble film with oral transmucosal fentanyl citrate. *Clin Drug Investig*. 2009;29:647-654.

104   Vasisht N, Gever LN, Tagarro I, Finn AL. Single-dose pharmacokinetics of fentanyl buccal soluble film. *Pain Med*. 2010;11:1017-1023.

105   Vasisht N, Stark J, Finn A. BEMA fentanyl shows a favorable pharmacokinetic profile and dose linearity in healthy volunteers. Presented at: Annual General Meeting of the American Society of Anesthesiologists; October 17, 2008; Orlando, FL.

106   Finn AL, Hill WC, Tagarro I, Gever LN. Absorption and tolerability of fentanyl buccal soluble film (FBSF) in patients with cancer in the presence of oral mucositis. *J Pain Res*. 2011;4:245-251.

107 Narang N, Sharma J. Sublingual mucosa as a route for systemic drug delivery. *Int J Pharm Pharm Sci.* 2011;3(Suppl 2):18-22.

108 Reynolds L, Geach J, Parikh N, Dillaha, L, Bull J. Safety and efficacy of fentanyl sublingual spray in the treatment of breakthrough cancer pain. Presented at: American Academy of Pain Medicine Annual Meeting; February 23–26, 2012; Palm Springs, CA.

109 Mercadante S, Radbruch L, Davies A, et al. A comparison of intranasal fentanyl spray with oral transmucosal fentanyl citrate for the treatment of breakthrough cancer pain: an open-label, randomised, crossover trial. *Curr Med Res Opin.* 2009;25:2805-2815.

110 Fine PG. Advances in cancer pain management. In: Lake CL, Rice IJ, Sperry RJ, eds. *Advances in Anesthesia.* St. Louis, Mo: Mosby-Year Book, Inc.;1995:145.

Chapter 4

Practical approach to the management of cancer breakthrough pain

Practical approach to the management of cancer breakthrough pain

Now that we have discussed the characteristics, definitions, and treatment of cancer breakthrough pain (cBTP), we will review a practical approach to managing cBTP through a step-by-step method, outlined by Mercadante and Davies (Figure 4.1) [1,2], and apply their recommended approaches through two case studies.

At the initiation of treatment and throughout treatment, the clinician and healthcare team should always tailor and individualize their treatment methods to the patient. The World Health Organization's (WHO's) pain ladder's recommendations of making the treatment of cBTP "for the individual" and with "attention to detail" are critical to remember when finding appropriate treatment options for the patient.

Step 1: Assessment of around-the-clock medication

After it is determined that a patient has cancer and pain flares, the clinician should then assess whether the patient's background pain is adequately controlled by an around-the-clock (ATC) medication. If a patient's background pain is well-controlled, they should report a pain score of 0–4 on the Numerical Rating Scale, where

D. R. Taylor., *Managing Cancer Breakthrough Pain*,
DOI: 10.1007/978-1-908517-83-8_4, © Springer Healthcare 2013

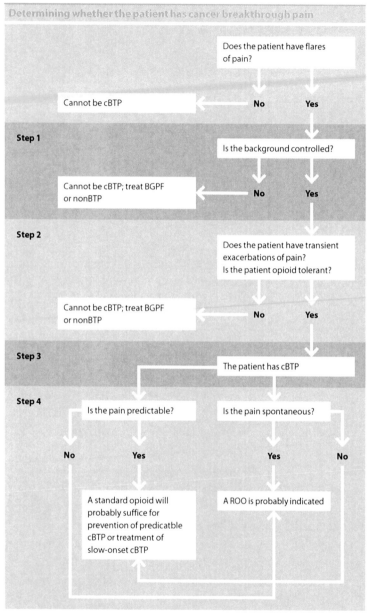

Figure 4.1 Determining whether the patient has cancer breakthrough pain. BGPF, background pain flare; BTP, breakthrough pain; cBTP cancer breakthrough pain; ROO, rapid-onset opioid. Data from Mercandante [1], Davies et al [2].

0 represents no pain and 10 represents the worst imaginable pain, for the majority of the day [2]; spikes or flares of pain should occur less than or equal to 5 times per day, on average 3–5 times per day. In most situations, if flares of pain are occurring more than 4 times per day then the physician should consider titration of the ATC medication; however, some patients may not tolerate increasing the ATC dose and might do better with more frequent cBTP medication dosing. Treatment should always be tailored to the patient's individual needs.

Step 2: Determination of opioid tolerance

Once the ATC medication has been optimally titrated to control the patient's background pain, then it must be determined if the patient is opioid tolerant. The US Food and Drug Administration (FDA) defines opioid tolerance to exist when the patient has been on an ATC opioid regimen equivalent to at least 60 mg of oral morphine daily, at least 25 µg of transdermal fentanyl per hour, at least 30 mg of oral oxycodone daily, at least 8 mg of oral hydromorphone daily, at least 25 mg oral oxymorphone daily, or an equianalgesic dose of another opioid daily for 1 week or longer (Table 3.3) [3–11]. If the patient meets these criteria, then they can be prescribed rapid-onset opioids (ROO) for the treatment of their cBTP [2].

Step 3: Treating cancer breakthrough pain

If the background pain is under adequate control, the patient is opioid tolerant, and episodes of pain require treatment with opioids, then the clinician and healthcare team should proceed to treat the patient's cBTP. The patient should be screened for aberrant drug behavior during initial examination, and their risk factors should be reviewed. The patient's recent history of behavior when using their ATC and rescue medications should be reviewed as well, and the clinician and healthcare team should take actions, if indicated, to address aberrant drug behavior. If the patient has been compliant with treatment, then opioids can be continued and the use of a ROO can be considered.

Step 4: Predictable or spontaneous?

The next step is to determine if a ROO is needed or whether standard opioids will suffice. This is best done by determining whether the patient's cBTP is predictable or spontaneous, and whether the pain has a rapidly escalating pattern or develops slowly from onset to peak intensity. If the pain is always predictable or if it is always slow to reach peak intensity (ie, it takes longer than 15 minutes to reach maximum intensity), then a standard opioid might be appropriate for use. The standard opioid can be given preemptively for predictable pain [12]. For spontaneous, slow-onset pain flares, a standard opioid may match the time course of the cBTP episode and could suffice. The ROOs are most helpful when the pain flares are unpredictable and/or rise rapidly to maximum intensity (ie, pain reaches maximum intensity in ≤15 minutes). Following the flow chart in Figure 4.1 is a simple technique that can help determine if a patient is having cBTP and whether it would best be managed with a standard opioid or a ROO [12].

Case studies

The following case studies use hypothetical patients to illustrate various aspects of cBTP management that might be encountered in clinical practice.

Assessing case study 1 for treatment management

Step 1: Assessment of background pain control

The patient reported good overall background pain control. The pain control was adequate for him to engage in the activities of daily living and to enjoy life; thus, this patient had adequately controlled background pain.

Step 2: Assessment of opioid tolerance

The patient was taking extended-release morphine at 60 mg/8 hours (or 180 mg/day). Since the background pain was controlled by an opioid (ie, morphine) at a dose of greater than or equal to 60 mg/day, and he had been on this dose for 1 week, the patient was considered opioid tolerant.

Step 3: Confirm that cancer breakthrough pain is present

The patient had well-controlled background pain and was opioid tolerant; he also had episodic flares of pain that broke through his background pain control. Thus, it was concluded that the patient had cBTP.

Step 4: Is the pain predictable?

The patient had reported that these flares of pain only occurred when he picked up his granddaughter. This is a type of incident, predictable pain. The pain described here is rapid in onset, but it is predictable. Therefore, pretreatment with a standard opioid will usually suffice for pain control [12]. At this point a regular-release opioid, such as oxycodone or morphine taken by the patient 30–60 minutes prior to visiting his granddaughter, might be prescribed [2,13].

However, other, nonpharmacologic strategies might also be tried. The patient could be instructed to avoid picking up his granddaughter by, for instance, sitting down in a chair to have his granddaughter climb to his lap. This might decrease the pain to the point where no medication is needed [2,13].

When the idea of using a preemptive analgesic was presented to the patient, he reported that sometimes when he picked up his granddaughter, he had minimal pain. He was concerned that if he took pain medication every time he went to see his granddaughter that he might become too sedated to enjoy the visit, especially if he did not need the opioid to counteract pain. In this situation, it was not possible to know which visits to pretreat. Due to this circumstance, the patient's cBTP can be considered incident-related and unpredictable [14].

Treatment options for case study 1

It was not possible to predict which incidents (eg, lifting the granddaughter) would result in pain and the patient had a reasonable concern about opioid effects unopposed by pain causing unwanted sedation. In this setting, the clinician has a number of different treatment options to offer the patient, some of which are:

1. Use of nonpharmacologic methods
2. Use of interventional techniques

3. Advising the patient to pretreat every time he was to have a visit with his granddaughter
4. Increasing the ATC medication to cover the cBTP
5. Advising the patient to stop lifting his granddaughter (eg, have her climb into his lap instead)
6. Allowing the patient to endure the pain
7. Use of a ROO to allow the patient to treat only the painful episodes

Nonpharmacologic treatment methods

A variety of nonpharmacological treatments have been reported to reduce pain. Some of these techniques include rubbing/massaging the pain site, application of heat or cold onto the site, distraction techniques, relaxation techniques, transcutaneous electrical nerve stimulation (TENS), and acupuncture [15,16]. There is little research to support that these techniques are helpful in treating cBTP, but this author has found them of benefit for some patients with noncancer incident pain. It is reasonable to try such techniques either before or alongside pharmacological therapy [2,15]. Patient 1 elected to try a TENS unit and thought that it was helpful, but it ultimately did not provide enough pain relief to eliminate the need for cBTP medication.

Interventional techniques

There are many interventional pain management techniques used for cancer pain management. Some of these include injection of neurolytic agents, such as alcohol or phenol onto nerves, plexus or intrathecally, radiofrequency techniques, vertebroplasty, percutaneous cordotomy, spinal cord stimulation, and others [17]. Interventional pain management techniques have not been studied in cBTP; however, interventional techniques have been helpful in the management of background cancer pain [16,18]. It is reasonable to think that interventional techniques that eliminate the majority or all of the background pain might improve cBTP if the cBTP is in the same location and of similar nature as the background pain. Thus, interventional techniques for pain management were considered in this patient.

A cervical percutaneous cordotomy was considered as the pain was unilateral and below the C5 dermatome level [18–20]. Results are generally good with this procedure and morbidity is low [19]. However, after the aggressive cancer treatment Patient 1 was not emotionally ready for further invasive treatments.

Numerous other interventional options could also have been considered. A few possible options would have been: intrathecal opioids and/or ziconotide [21], intrathecal or epidural neurolysis [22], and spinal cord stimulation [23].

In some patients, interventional techniques can be used as sole agents for the control of cancer pain or as useful adjuncts to supplement analgesia provided by medications [23,24]. The maximal benefit from interventional procedures is likely to occur when they are performed in appropriately selected patients early in treatment [23,25]. Neurolytic procedures should be considered prior to initiation of high-dose narcotic therapy, palliative radiation, chemotherapy, or surgery when possible [23].

Pretreatment

Patient 1 could have been pretreated with a regular-release opioid prior to every visit with his granddaughter, but since he did not have cBTP episodes at every incident, he was concerned about unwanted sedation, nausea, dizziness, or other opioid side effects [13]. For these reasons, it was decided not to pretreat every episode.

Since the time-to-peak effect of oral morphine and oxycodone is approximately 1 hour [26,27], these drugs are not well suited for unpredictable pain that escalates to maximum intensity in minutes; pretreatment with these medications should be done at least 30 minutes and sometimes 60 minutes prior to the incident [2,12].

Increasing the background pain medication

Increasing the ATC medication used to treat background pain could have been considered. One study of patients with metastatic bone disease found that increasing the ATC medication to above the level that was needed to control background pain did allow a significant number of patients to achieve adequate cBTP control with an acceptable level of side effects; however, nausea, vomiting, and drowsiness developed in some patients and necessitated a dose reduction. This study was not blinded and lacked a control group so its results need to be interpreted with caution [28]. However, this study does suggest that, for some patients, increasing the ATC medication might be an option for controlling cBTP episodes [15]. This patient chose not to increase his ATC medication because he had adequate control of background pain, and he did not want to risk being overly sedated so he would not be able to enjoy his time with his granddaughter.

Modifying the circumstances

Sometimes the patients can modify their behavior to prevent or reduce cBTP episodes. For example, in this case, the patient might have sat in a chair and allowed his granddaughter to climb into his lap instead of picking her up, thus avoiding an incident that may induce a cBTP episode. This might have reduced or eliminated his need for cBTP medication [2,13]. The patient agreed to try this strategy. He found that while there did seem to be some benefit from modifying the circumstances under which his cBTP occurred, this approach did not completely eliminate the need for cBTP medication.

Enduring the pain

Some patients do not see the need to treat every cBTP episode and, based on the patient's wishes, no treatment may be what the patient desires. Even patients prescribed medication for cBTP may not use it to treat every cBTP episode. One observational study of oncology patients' utilization of breakthrough pain medications found that the majority of patients (77% of prescribed study population) did not take cBTP medication every time they experience cBTP, often because the cBTP episode was of minimal intensity, short in duration, or sometimes they did not medicate themselves because of concerns about opioid side effects, such as sedation or nausea [29]. If the patient has a rational reason for not taking cBTP medication, then letting the patient endure their pain, and essentially do nothing, is a reasonable option. If the reasons for not taking the cBTP medication appear irrational to the clinician, then patient education should help the patient make better choices [29].

Patient 1 was offered the option of not receiving treatment for the cBTP; however, he did not elect to pursue this option. Furthermore, he understood that it would always be his choice whether to treat an episode of cBTP with the cBTP medication or not.

Treatment with a rapid-onset opioid

With a ROO the patient can take the medication with him every time he visits with his granddaughter and to use it if he needs it. The rapid onset of pain relief with the ROO will mean that he does not have to suffer for a prolonged period if a pain episode should occur. Knowing that the patient will have an effective medication if a pain episode should occur might reduce anxiety about having pain, which in itself may reduce the overall pain experience [30]. Feeling more in control of the situation may lessen anxiety and hence lessen pain [31–35]. Patient 1 was interested in using a ROO.

Treatment of case study 1

Once all the above treatment options had been explained to the patient, and risk and benefits of each option are discussed, the patient decided to use a ROO. When assessing a patient for ROO treatment, the temporal profile of the cBTP episodes should be evaluated so the appropriate agent can be prescribed; the agent's "time to meaningful pain relief" should match the pain onset, peak intensity time, and duration [36].

Before prescribing a ROO, the clinician and patient discussed the risks of his granddaughter accidentally taking the ROO or other medications. Accidental ingestion of a ROO or ATC medication dose could be fatal to a child and might also be fatal to a nonopioid tolerant adult as well [37]. Many of the drugs that are abused are medications prescribed for other family members, so all patients on opioids who will be around children of any age should be counseled about the safe storage of medications [38]. It is prudent for patients to use some form of lockable container to secure all of their medications [39].

Patient 1 was started on a ROO and this was titrated to effect. During this process monitoring for side effects and aberrant drug behavior was carried out. His ATC medication was maintained at the previously determined effective dose. After titrating the ROO over several days, an effective dose was found and the patient did well.

Case study 2

Patient 2 is a 45-year-old woman with breast cancer who had a mastectomy 12 months prior to a local chest wall recurrence with metastases to the ribs and spine. The disease had progressed despite aggressive treatment and the patient had exhausted all chemotherapeutic and nuclear medicine interventions that were deemed reasonable. Her background pain was treated with transdermal fentanyl at 75 μg/hour with patches being changed every 72 hours. She was on a short-acting opioid (SAO) for "pain flares". The patient's major concern was to remain functional as a mother to her teenage children as long as possible while on treatment. Thus, she wanted to control her pain with as little sedation as possible.

She reported three different types of pain flares. First, she had "shooting", "electrical" pains in her chest wall that were associated with the locally invasive cancer. These shooting pains seemed to travel from the front and around to the back of her chest wall, and she reported numbness in the anterior chest wall in the area of pain. This pain and numbness were in a dermatomal distribution, and were unpredictable. They reached maximum intensity in seconds and lasted for seconds to minutes at most. They occurred at any time of day and sometimes occurred on and off all day long. This pain had not changed significantly with the transdermal fentanyl.

Second, she had back pain if she stood or walked too long. This axial spine pain was consistent in location with her vertebral body metastatic disease. It was primarily dull and aching, although with activity it could be sharp and severe. It occurred primarily with activity. This pain had improved significantly with the transdermal fentanyl. Reflexes and sensory exams were normal in all extremities; toes were down-going (negative Babinski's sign) and there had been no changes in bowel or bladder control/function. While this back pain had been helped significantly by the transdermal fentanyl, she did report that the back pain got predictably worse the third day after application of a transdermal fentanyl patch. On those days the back pain would occur even when she was at rest. These episodic increases in pain lasted from 12 to 24 hours and improved only after a new transdermal fentanyl patch was applied.

Her third type of pain flare was an unpredictable chest wall pain that was different from the electrical, shooting pain. It had knife-like, stabbing, and aching components. This pain was sometimes related to movement or deep breathing but occurred at other times for no apparent reason, and was spontaneous. It had a nondermatomal distribution. When it occurred it started suddenly, reached maximum intensity in minutes, and lasted for 30 minutes to an hour. These pain episodes occurred no more than 2 or 3 times per day. This pain was also helped to some extent by the transdermal fentanyl.

Practically managing case study 2
Step 1: Assessment of background pain control
This patient had adequately controlled background pain most of the time, but on the third day after application of a transdermal fentanyl the pain predictably increased. This represents end-of-dose failure, and needed to be addressed by either increasing the dose of the transdermal fentanyl or by decreasing the dosing interval to 48 hours [7]. Some authors list "end-of-dose" or "end-of-dose failure" as a fourth type of cBTP; however, other authors, including myself, do not consider end-of-dose failure as a true type of cBTP, as the pain is not flaring up but rather the analgesic level is falling. End-of-dose failure is treated by correcting the ATC medication dosing rather than by adding a cBTP medication [15].

Some patients, like Patient 2, will report episodic increases in pain that last more than a couple of hours; while this has been reported and studied, it is unusual [40]. It is prudent to reevaluate patients with long episodes of cBTP to make sure that this pain is not really a background pain flare (BGPF) or end-of-dose failure as with Patient 2. Patients with unusually long episodes of cBTP may require further titration of their ATC basal analgesic. The clinician should always be prepared to reassess the patient and the treatment plan to tailor and individualize the patient's treatment appropriately to their needs [2]; this is another example of falling back on the basic WHO principles of making the treatment plan effective "for the individual" and with "attention to detail".

The transdermal fentanyl dose was changed to 75 µg/hour every 48 hours. This corrected the end-of-dose failure. In this patient, correction of the end-of-dose failure was undertaken first to ensure adequate background pain control. Then the patient was reassessed for cBTP.

Reassessment
After the adjustment of the transdermal fentanyl dose, the patient had adequately controlled background pain; however, the patient continued to report unpredictable chest wall pain and incident-related back pain.

Step 2: Assessment of opioid tolerance
The patient had been on 75 µg/hour transdermal fentanyl for more than 1 week; therefore, she was considered to be opioid tolerant.

Step 3: Confirm that cancer breakthrough pain is present
The patient had flares of pain in the setting of adequately controlled background pain and was opioid tolerant; therefore, the patient had cBTP.

Step 4: Is the pain predictable?
Patient 2 had flares of electrical, shooting pains in her chest wall with associated numbness, consistent with tumor invasion of an intercostal nerve. This neuropathic pain was spontaneous and unpredictable. Her back pain was incident-related and predictable. The patient also had unpredictable, spontaneous chest wall pain that was not dermatomal in distribution and which had responded somewhat to the transdermal fentanyl.

Treatment options for case study 2
Although neuropathic pain can be managed by opioids (eg, by increasing the ATC opioid) [41,42], painful dysesthesias (described here as electrical or shooting pain and numbness) may respond more effectively to an anticonvulsant drug [43,44]. The anticonvulsant can be started at a low dose to minimize the risk of sedation and titrated to effect. The patient

was started on an anticonvulsant with improvement in the shooting and electrical cBTP episodes.

Pain from neoplastic invasion of an intercostal nerve can also be treated with a variety of interventional techniques, such as percutaneous radiofrequency neurectomy [45], neurolytic intercostal nerve blocks [46], or intrathecal neurolytic block [47]. These interventional approaches to pain management can be considered if unwanted side effects occur from oral agents [25].

The back pain was incident-related and predictable, so an SAO could have been administered 30–45 minutes prior to anticipated activities to manage this pain [2,12]; however, the patient could also have been considered a candidate for vertebroplasty [48,49] for the vertebral metastatic disease. As the patient had expressed the desire for treatment with minimal sedation, such an interventional approach may reduce the need for systemic analgesics and reduce the risk of sedation. It is important for the clinician not to solely focus on pharmacologic management to the exclusion of other methods of cancer pain management [50].

The patient's chest-wall pain, which was not dermatomal in distribution and therefore, probably somatic rather than neuropathic in nature, could be expected to respond well to an opioid and had previously responded partially to the transdermal fentanyl patch. Therefore, the patient could be treated with a ROO as the chest wall cBTP qualified as unpredictable and spontaneous cBTP [2,12].

Drug abuse by family members

Many of the drugs abused by illicit users come from medications prescribed for other family members [38]; since Patient 2 has teenage children who could accidentally or purposefully take her opioid medications, she should be counseled regarding the safe storage of her medications. While the mother may protest that there is no need to be concerned about her children, it is better for the clinician, and thus the patient, to err on the side of caution and to have a discussion regarding the drugs and aberrant behavior [38]. As noted in case study 1, it is always prudent for patients to use some form of lockable container to secure all of their medications [39].

Treatment for case study 2

The patient was started on a ROO for the spontaneous cBTP and an SAO, 30–60 minutes before activity, for the predictable cBTP. These were individually titrated to effect [2,51]. The ATC basal medication was maintained (transdermal fentanyl 75-µg/hour patch changed every 48 hours), and her background pain was adequately controlled. She was also referred for a vertebroplasty [50]. This procedure controlled the back pain and at this point the SAO was discontinued. The anticonvulsant controlled the dysesthetic pain. A ROO managed the spontaneous, rapidly onsetting cBTP, the long-acting opioid (transdermal fentanyl) controlled her background pain, the vertebroplasty eliminated her back pain, and an anticonvulsant managed her dysesthetic pain. With improved pain control the patient could move and walk better, and ultimately she was more actively involved with her children. This pain management approach helped the patient with the combined goals of improving function, controlling pain, and minimizing sedation.

References

1 Mercadante S. Managing breakthrough pain. *Curr Pain Headache Rep.* 2011;15:244-249.
2 Davies AN, Dickman A, Reid C, Stevens AM, Zeppetella G; Science Committee of the Association for Palliative Medicine of Great Britain and Ireland. The management of cancer-related breakthrough pain: recommendations of a task group of the Science Committee of the Association for Palliative Medicine of Great Britain and Ireland. *Eur J Pain.* 2009;13:331-338.
3 Avinza [package insert]. Bristol, TN: King Pharmaceuticals, Inc.; 2012.
4 Embeda [package insert]. Piscataway Township, NJ: Alpharma Pharmaceuticals LLC; 2009.
5 Kadian [package insert]. Morristown, NJ: Actavis Elizabeth LLC; 2012.
6 MS Contin [package insert]. Stamford, CT: Purdue Pharma L.P.; 2009.
7 Duragesic [package insert]. Titusville, NJ: Janssen Pharmaceuticals, Inc.; 2012.
8 OxyContin [package insert]. Stamford, CT: Purdue Pharma L.P.; 2010.
9 Palladone [package insert]. Stamford, CT: Purdue Pharma L.P.; 2006.
10 Exalgo [package insert]. Hazelwood, MO: Mallinckrodt LLC; 2012.
11 Opana ER [package insert]. Chadds Ford, PA: Endo Pharmaceuticals Inc.; 2012.
12 Bennett D, Burton AW, Fishman S, et al. Consensus panel recommendations for the assessment and management of breakthrough pain: Part 2 Management. *P T.* 2005;30:354-361.
13 McCarberg BH. The treatment of breakthrough pain. *Pain Med.* 2007;8(Suppl 1):S8-S13.
14 Bennett D, Burton AW, Fishman S, et al. Consensus panel recommendations for the assessment and management of breakthrough pain: Part 1 Assessment. *P T.* 2005;30:296-301.
15 Zeppetella G. Breakthrough pain in cancer patients. *Clin Oncol (R Coll Radiol).* 2011;23:393-398.
16 Tay W, Ho KY. The role of interventional therapies in cancer pain management. *Ann Acad Med Singapore.* 2009;38:989-997.
17 Bhaskar AK. Interventional management of cancer pain. *Curr Opin Support Palliat Care.* 2012;6:1-9.

18 Vissers KC, Besse K, Wagemans M, et al. Pain in patients with cancer. *Pain Pract.* 2011;11:453-475.

19 Zuurmond WW, Perez RS, Loer SA. Role of cervical cordotomy and other neurolytic procedures in thoracic cancer pain. *Curr Opin Support Palliat Care.* 2010;4:6-10.

20 Bekar A, Kocaeli H, Abaş F, Bozkurt M. Bilateral high-level percutaneous cervical cordotomy in cancer pain due to lung cancer: a case report. *Surg Neurol.* 2007;67:504-507.

21 Alicino I, Giglio M, Manca F, Bruno F, Puntillo F. Intrathecal combination of ziconotide and morphine for refractory cancer pain: a rapidly acting and effective choice. *Pain.* 2012;153:245-249.

22 Takahashi-Sato K, Hashimoto K, et al. Two cases of thoracic epidural neurolysis after local anesthetic titration in cancer patients. *Fukushima J Med Sci.* 2011;57:66-68.

23 Arter OE, Racz GB. Pain management of the oncologic patient. *Semin Surg Oncol.* 1990;6:162-172.

24 Miguel R. Interventional treatment of cancer pain: the fourth step in the World Health Organization analgesic ladder? *Cancer Control.* 2000;7:149-156.

25 Patt RB, Jain S. Therapeutic decision making for invasive procedures. In Patt RB, ed. *Cancer Pain.* Philadelphia, PA: J.B. Lippincott Company; 1993:275-284.

26 Collins SL, Faura CC, Moore RA, McQuay HJ. Peak plasma concentrations after oral morphine: a systematic review. *J Pain Symptom Manage.* 1998;16:388-402.

27 Poyhia R, Seppala T, Olkkola KT, Kalso E. The pharmacokinetics and metabolism of oxycodone after intramuscular and oral administration to healthy subjects. *Br J Clin Pharmacol.* 1992;33:617-621.

28 Mercadante S, Villari P, Ferrera P, Casuccio A. Optimization of opioid therapy for preventing incident pain associated with bone metastases. J *Pain Symptom Manage.* 2004;28:505-510.

29 Davies AN, Vriens J, Kennett A, McTaggart M. An observational study of oncology patients' utilization of breakthrough pain medication. *J Pain Symptom Manage.* 2008;35:406-411.

30 Hill HE, Kornetsky CH, Flanary HG, Wikler A. Effects of anxiety and morphine on discrimination of intensities of painful stimuli. *J Clin Invest.* 1952;31:473-480.

31 Crisson JE, Keefe FJ. The relationship of locus of control to pain coping strategies and psychological distress in chronic pain patients. *Pain.* 1988;35:147-154.

32 Sternbach RA. Psychophysiology of pain. *Int J Psychiatry Med.* 1975;6:63-73.

33 Chapman CR. Psychological aspects of pain patient treatment. *Arch Surg.* 1977;112:767-772.

34 Clum GA, Luscomb RL, Scott L. Relaxation training and cognitive redirection strategies in the treatment of acute pain. *Pain.* 1982;12:175-183.

35 Taenzer P, Melzack R, Jeans ME. Influence of psychological factors on postoperative pain, mood and analgesic requirements. *Pain.* 1986;24:331-342.

36 Zeppetella G. Opioids for cancer breakthrough pain: a pilot study reporting patient assessment of time to meaningful pain relief. *J Pain Symptom Manage.* 2008;35:563-567.

37 TIRF REMS ACCESS. TIRF REMS Access Program Home. What is the TIRF REMS Access Program? www.tirfremsaccess.com. Accessed February 1, 2013.

38 Hardesty C. Friends and family are primary sources of abused prescription drugs. Office of National Drug Control Policy. www.whitehouse.gov/blog/2012/04/25/friends-and-family-are-primary-sources-abused-prescription-drugs. Published April 25, 2012. Accessed February 1, 2013.

39 Storing medicine safely. MedlinePlus. www.nlm.nih.gov/medlineplus/ency/article/007189.htm. Updated March 26, 2011. Accessed February 1, 2013.

40 Mercadante S, Zagonel V, Breda E, et al. Breakthrough pain in oncology: a longitudinal study. *J Pain Symptom Manage.* 2010;40:183-190.

41 Rowbotham MC, Twilling L, Davies PS, Reisner L, Taylor K, Mohr D. Oral opioid therapy for chronic peripheral and central neuropathic pain. *N Engl J Med.* 2003;348:1223-1232.

42 Eisenberg E, McNicol E, Carr DB. Opioids for neuropathic pain. *Cochrane Database Syst Rev.* 2006;(3):CD006146.

43 Chaparro LE, Wiffen PJ, Moore RA, Gilron I. Combination pharmacotherapy for the treatment of neuropathic pain in adults. *Cochrane Database Syst Rev*. 2012;7:CD008943.

44 Eisenberg E, Peterson D. Neuropathic Pain Pharmacotherapy. In: Fishman SM, Ballantyne JC, Rathmell JP, eds. *Bonica's Management of Pain*. 4th ed. New York, NY: Lippincott Williams & Wilkins; 2010:1194-1207.

45 Tasker RB. Neurosurgical and neuroaugmentative intervention. In: Patt RB, ed. *Cancer Pain*. Philadelphia, PA: J.B. Lippincott Company; 1993:471-500.

46 Patt RB. Peripheral neurolysis and the management of cancer pain. In: Patt RB, ed. *Cancer Pain*. Philadelphia, PA: J.B. Lippincott Company; 1993:359-376.

47 Swerdlow M. Neurolytic blocks of the neuraxis. In: Patt RB, ed. *Cancer Pain*. Philadelphia, PA: J.B. Lippincott Company; 1993:427-442.

48 Martin JB, Wetzel SG, Seium Y, et al. Percutaneous vertebroplasty in metastatic disease: transpedicular access and treatment of lysed pedicles—initial experience. *Radiology*. 2003;229:593-597.

49 Pilitsis JG, Rengachary SS. The role of vertebroplasty in metastatic spinal disease. *Neurosurg Focus*. 2001;11:e9.

50 Picot T, Hamid B. Decision-making in the cancer pain setting: Beyond the WHO ladder. *Tech Reg Anesth Pain Manag*. 2010;14:19-24.

51 Portenoy RK. Treatment of cancer pain. *Lancet*. 2011;377:2236-2247.

Abuse, aberrant drug behavior, diversion, and addiction

There is growing concern about abuse, aberrant drug behavior, diversion, and addiction in patients with cancer who are treated with opioids [1]. Patients with cancer are surviving longer and acute cancer pain is often transformed into a chronic cancer pain syndrome [2], with an increased risk of abuse and addiction [3].

Definitions

Abuse is the use of an illicit drug or the intentional self-administration of a prescription (or over-the-counter) medication for any nonmedical purpose, such as altering one's state of consciousness (eg, "getting high") [4]. Aberrant drug behavior is any medication-related behaviors that depart from strict adherence to the prescribed therapeutic plan-of-care [4]. Diversion is the intentional removal of a medication from legitimate distribution and dispensing channels. Diversion also involves the sharing or purchasing of prescription medication between family members and friends, or individual theft from family and friends [4]. Addiction is a primary, chronic disease of the brain's reward, motivation, memory, and related circuitry. Dysfunction in these circuits leads to characteristic biological, psychological, social, and spiritual manifestations [4].

Patients at risk

This author has found in clinical practice that the use of rapid-onset opioids (ROO), SAOs, and LAOs for cancer pain have all been associated with

D. R. Taylor., *Managing Cancer Breakthrough Pain*, DOI: 10.1007/978-1-908517-83-8_5, © Springer Healthcare 2013 diversion and aberrant drug-related behaviors [5,6]. The overall lifetime prevalence of abuse and addiction developing in the general population is 6.2% [7]. It is likely that a similar proportion of patients with cancer will be at-risk for developing abuse and/or addiction. Physicians treating cancer pain must learn to employ the tools that are routine in the management of chronic noncancer pain [8,9], such as:

- screening for risk of aberrant drug behavior prior to initiating opioid treatment;
- consulting prescription monitoring programs;
- conducting urine drug testing, which evaluates the patient for the presence or absence of drugs that are prescribed, unprescribed, and/or illicit;
- requiring that patients use opioid consent forms that defines the risk of chronic opioid therapy; and
- having the patient sign an opioid agreement that defines the patient's responsibility with regard to opioid use.

It is important to monitor all patients prescribed long-term opioids since there is no definitive screening test to predict which patients will develop aberrant behavior or addiction when treated with opioids [9]. In the author's opinion, all patients receiving long-term opioid therapy should be monitored with random urine, saliva, or blood toxicology testing to help ensure compliance with their opioid regimen. Use of these tools can help detect aberrant drug behavior and diversion. A recent panel of experts reviewed the literature on urine drug testing, and recommended that all patients who are prescribed opioids for more than 3 months should be tested [10]. In effect, all patients should be considered "at risk".

Physicians prescribing opioids for cancer pain have a responsibility to help prevent diversion as well as abuse and addiction. The current epidemic of prescription-drug abuse has lead to an increase of accidental prescription drug overdoses and deaths. Currently, at the time of publication, deaths caused by prescription-drug overdoses have become the number one cause of accidental death in the United States, exceeding the number of accidental deaths from car accidents [11]. Understanding which patients are at high risk for abuse and/or diversion can help practitioners target monitoring procedures, such as the frequency of urine drug tests and pill counts, and it is hoped that such monitoring coupled with appropriate interventions may help reduce the number of accidental drug overdose deaths. It is highly recommended that all patients with cancer placed on long-term opioid therapy be assessed for the risk of abuse and diversion prior to initiating opioid therapy so that monitoring can be tailored to their respective risk level [3].

More than 3 out of 4 people who misuse prescription analgesics use drugs that were prescribed to someone else [12]. About 5% of these nonmedical drug users took the drugs from a friend or relative without asking. In over 20 years of experience, this author has seen a number of cases of diversion by patients or family members of patients with cancer. Thus, the prescriber must consider diversion by friends and family as well as the patient in their overall risk assessment for prescribing opioids to the patient.

Some groups who are particularly at-risk for prescription-drug addiction, abuse, diversion, and overdose are those who:

- Obtain multiple controlled-substance prescriptions from multiple providers, which is a practice known as "doctor shopping" [13,14].
- Take high daily dosages of prescription painkillers and those who misuse multiple abuse-prone prescription drugs [14–18].
- Have lower incomes and live in rural areas [19].
- Are on Medicaid.
    - People on Medicaid are prescribed painkillers at twice the rate of non-Medicaid patients and are at six times the risk of prescription pain medication overdose [20,21]. One study from Washington State found that 45% of people who died from prescription pain medication overdoses were Medicaid enrollees [20].
- Have mental illness and those with a history of substance abuse [18].
    - The rapid onset of the ROOs make them useful for treating cBTP, but also attractive to drug abusers. Patients with a history of drug abuse, impulsive behavior, or who tend to become panicky or desperate in the face of their pain, are not good candidates for ROOs [22].

Screening prior to initiating a rapid-onset opioid

When ROO treatment is initiated, it is assumed that the patient is already on an around-the-clock (ATC) opioid for basal analgesia. In this scenario, the patient should already have had a routine history, physical examinations and screening for opioid therapy, which would include inspection of the skin for needle tracks, scars from "skin popping", and abnormalities of the nasal septum from cocaine use as well as any history of previous licit and illicit drug use. Routine, random urine drug screens should have been established and screening tools should have been administered; some screening tools include the Screener and Opioid Assessment for Patients with Pain-Revised (SOAPP-R) [23] or Opioid Risk Tool (ORT) [22,24], which are "paper and pen" screening questionnaires filled out by the patient that assess risk of aberrant drug behavior. Thus, before prescribing a ROO, screening for the risk of aberrant drug behavior should have been completed and be available for review. Reviewing the patient's screening results and examination notes is critical to be able to appropriately treat the patient's cBTP episodes. For example, if the patient is thought to be at-risk for developing aberrant drug behavior, prior to initiating treatment with a ROO, it would be highly recommended for the patient to consult with a pain and addiction specialist; if this is not possible, then follow-up visits should be scheduled every 1 or 2 weeks until the patient is deemed stable.

In addition to examinations and screenings, the clinician and health-care team can also monitor proper drug use by having an open-line of communication with family members and caregivers, and by counting dosage units. Having the patient return used bottles, blister packs, and/or oral transmucosal fentanyl citrate handles for counting can help monitor for drug overuse and diversion.

A number of features suggestive of aberrant opioid-related behavior have been described and are listed in Table 5.1 [25]. These should be considered "yellow flags" and the prescriber should proceed with caution should any of these behaviors occur during treatment; however, there is not one yellow flag that leads to the diagnosis of drug abuse or addiction but these events should be considered as prompts for the clinician to reassess the patient for the possibility of emerging addiction. If abuse

Features suggestive of aberrant opioid-related behavior
Unexpected results on toxicologic screening
Frequent requests for dose increase
Concurrent use of a nonprescription psychoactive substance
Failure to follow dosage schedule
Failure to adhere to concurrently recommended treatments
Frequently reported loss of prescriptions or medications
Frequent visits to the emergency department for opioid therapy
Missed follow-up visits
Frequent extra appointments at the clinic or office
Prescriptions obtained from a second provider
Tampering with prescriptions

Table 5.1 Features suggestive of aberrant opioid-related behavior. Data from Ballantyne et al [25].

or addiction is suspected, then these problems must be treated concurrently with the cancer pain. Consultation with an addiction medicine physician is recommended [8].

References

1   Koyyalagunta D, Burton AW, Toro MP, Driver L, Novy DM. Opioid abuse in cancer pain: report of two cases and presentation of an algorithm of multidisciplinary care. *Pain Physician.* 2011;14:E361-E371.

2   Paice JA. Chronic treatment-related pain in cancer survivors. *Pain.* 2011;152(3 Suppl):S84-S89.

3   Burton AW, Fine PG, Passik SD. Transformation of acute cancer pain to chronic cancer pain syndromes. *J Support Oncol.* 2012;10:89-95.

4   Corsini E, Zacharoff KL. Definitions related to aberrant drug-related behavior: Is there correct terminology? PainEdu.org. www.painedu.org/articles_timely.asp?ArticleNumber=58. Published October 29, 2011. Accessed February 1, 2013.

5   Núñez-Olarte JM, Álvarez-Jiménez P. Emerging opioid abuse in terminal cancer patients taking oral transmucosal fentanyl citrate for breakthrough pain. *J Pain Symptom Manage.* 2011;42:e6-e8.

6   Passik SD, Messina J, Golsorkhi A, Xie F. Aberrant drug-related behavior observed during clinical studies involving patients taking chronic opioid therapy for persistent pain and fentanyl buccal tablet for breakthrough pain. *J Pain Symptom Manage.* 2010 Jun 24. [Epub ahead of print].

7   Ries RK, Fiellin DA, Miller SC, Saitz R. *Principles of Addiction Medicine.* 4th Ed. Philadelphia, PA: Lippincott Williams & Wilkins; 2009.

8   Kircher S, Zacny J, Apfelbaum SM, et al. Understanding and treating opioid addiction in a patient with cancer pain. *J Pain.* 2011;12:1025-1031.

9   Gourlay, DL, Heit HA, Almahrezi A. Universal precautions in pain medicine: a rational approach to the treatment of chronic pain. *Pain Med.* 2005;6:107-112.

10 Couto JE, Peppin JF, Fine PG, Passik SD, Goldfarb NI. Developing recommendations for urine drug monitoring for patients on long-term opioid therapy. Presented at: The 2012 AAPM Annual Meeting; February 26, 2012; Palm Springs, CA.

11 Warner M, Chen LH, Makuc DM, Anderson RN, Miniño AM. Drug poisoning deaths in the United States, 1980–2008. *NCHS Data Brief*. 2011;81:1-8.

12 US Department of Health and Human Services. Results from the 2010 National Survey on Drug Use and Health: Mental Health Findings. www.cdc.gov/nchs/data/databriefs/db81.pdf. Published January 2012. Accessed February 1, 2013.

13 White AG, Birnbaum HG, Schiller M, Tang J, Katz NP. Analytic models to identify patients at risk for prescription opioid abuse. *Am J Managed Care*. 2009;15:897-906.

14 Hall AJ, Logan JE, Toblin RL, et al. Patterns of abuse among unintentional pharmaceutical overdose fatalities. *JAMA*. 2008;300:2613-2620.

15 Green TC, Graub LE, Carver HW, Kinzly M, Heimer R. Epidemiologic trends and geographic patterns of fatal opioid intoxications in Connecticut, USA: 1997–2007. *Drug Alcohol Depend*. 2011;115:221-228.

16 Paulozzi LJ, Logan JE, Hall AJ, McKinstry E, Kaplan JA, Crosby AE. A comparison of drug overdose deaths involving methadone and other opioid analgesics in West Virginia. *Addiction*. 2009;104:1541-1548.

17 Dunn KM, Saunders KW, Rutter CM, et al. Opioid prescriptions for chronic pain and overdose: a cohort study. *Ann Intern Med*. 2010;152:85-92.

18 Bohnert AS, Valenstein M, Bair MJ, et al. Association between opioid prescribing patterns and opioid overdose-related deaths. *JAMA*. 2011;305:1315-1321.

19 Centers for Disease Control and Prevention. CDC Grand Rounds: Prescription Drug Overdoses – a US Epidemic. *MMWR*. 2012;61:10-13.

20 Centers for Disease Control and Prevention. Overdose deaths involving prescription opioids among Medicaid enrollees – Washington, 2004–2007. MMWR. 2009;58;1171-1175.

21 Braden JB, Fan MY, Edlund MJ, Martin BC, DeVries A, Sullivan MD. Trends in use of opioids by noncancer pain type 2000-2005 among Arkansas Medicaid and HealthCore enrollees: results from the TROUP study. *J Pain*. 2008;9:1026-1035.

22 Starr TD, Rogak LJ, Passik SD. Substance abuse in cancer pain. *Curr Pain Headache Rep*. 2010;14:268-275.

23 SOAPP-R. OpioidRisk. www.opioidrisk.com/node/1209. Accessed February 1, 2013.

24 ORT. OpioidRisk. www.opioidrisk.com/node/1203. Accessed February 1, 2013.

25 Ballantyne JC, Mao J. Opioid therapy for chronic pain. *N Engl J Med*. 2003;349:1943-1953.

Chapter 6

TIRF REMS Access program

What are REMS and TIRF REMS?

A Risk Evaluation and Mitigation Strategies (REMS) program is a risk management plan that uses risk minimization strategies beyond approved drug labeling to manage serious risks associated with a medication. Under the US Food and Drug Administration (FDA) Amendments Act of 2007, the FDA has the authority to require a manufacturer to develop a REMS program when the FDA finds it is necessary to ensure that the benefits of a drug outweigh its risks, and to help ensure safe use of the medication. A REMS plan can include a medication guide or patient package insert, communication plan, or one or more of these elements to assure safe use. Also, an implementation system and a timetable for submission of the REMS assessments may also be delineated in the REMS program for any particular drug [1]. These regulations only apply to drugs used in the United States.

REMS are developed by drug manufacturers and approved by the FDA. The FDA has required that all rapid-onset opioids (ROOs) have a REMS program. Initially, every ROO had a different REMS program but more recently one REMS program has been developed for all of the currently available ROOs in the United States:

- ABSTRAL® (fentanyl) sublingual tablets;
- ACTIQ® (fentanyl citrate) oral transmucosal lozenge;
- FENTORA® (fentanyl citrate) buccal tablet;
- LAZANDA® (fentanyl) nasal spray;

D. R. Taylor., *Managing Cancer Breakthrough Pain*,
DOI: 10.1007/978-1-908517-83-8_6, © Springer Healthcare 2013

- ONSOLIS® fentanyl buccal soluble film;
- SUBSYS™ fentanyl sublingual spray; and
- generic equivalents of these drugs.

The FDA approved a shared, single-system REMS for transmucosal immediate release fentanyl (TIRF) medicines to reduce the burden on the healthcare system of having separate REMS programs in place for individual TIRF medicines. Prescribers, pharmacies, distributors, and outpatients will only need to enroll in the TIRF REMS Access program to be able to prescribe, dispense, or receive all drugs in the TIRF medicines class [1].

What are the goals of the TIRF REMS Access program?

The goals of the TIRF REMS Access program are to mitigate the risk of misuse, abuse, addiction, overdose, and serious complications due to medication errors [2]. The patient, the physician, and the pharmacist are all required to complete educational materials and registries prior to prescribing (for the physician), receiving (for the patient), and dispensing (for the pharmacist) a ROO. Physicians must complete a knowledge assessment on the ROO's prescribing information, and pharmacists must complete a similar assessment on dispensing a ROO. The pharmacist is required to register to ensure that they understand the safe use of ROOs and so that they may answer patient questions and reinforce patient education regarding safe use and storage of this class of opioids. Wholesalers and distributors of ROOs must also register and agree to distribute ROOs only to registered pharmacists. Inpatient use (hospital, hospice, nursing home) of ROOs is exempt from the TIRF REMS Access program requirement.

The TIRF REMS Access program requirements are meant to ensure that prescribers have received education on the safe use of ROOs prior to prescribing and patients are counseled on safe-use of the ROOs prior to receiving a prescription. To support the latter, patients and physicians must sign a Patient–Prescriber Agreement Form that reviews the safe use of these drugs and this form must be kept in the patient's chart. Complete information about the TIRF REMS Access program can be found at www.TIRFREMSaccess.com [2]. Prescribers must reenroll every 2 years.

Efforts to enhance patient safety

The TIRF REMS Access program focuses on the following [2]:

1. TIRF medicines can be abused in a manner similar to other opioid agonists, legal or illicit. Consider the potential for abuse when prescribing or dispensing TIRF medicines in situations where the physician or pharmacist is concerned about an increased risk of misuse, abuse, or diversion.

2. Serious adverse events, including deaths, in patients treated with some oral transmucosal fentanyl medicines have been reported. Deaths occurred as a result of improper patient selection (eg, use in opioid-nontolerant patients) and/or improper dosing. The substitution of a TIRF medicine for any other fentanyl medicine, including another TIRF medicine, may result in fatal overdose.

3. TIRF medicines are indicated only for the management of breakthrough pain in adult (18 years of age or older, or 16 years of age or older for ACTIQ® brand and generic equivalents) patients with cancer who are already receiving and who are tolerant to around-the-clock (ATC) opioid therapy for their underlying persistent cancer pain [3].

4. Patients considered opioid tolerant are those who are taking the following daily opioid dose for 1 week or longer:
   - at least 60 mg of oral morphine/daily;
   - at least 25 µg transdermal fentanyl/hour;
   - at least 30 mg of oral oxycodone daily;
   - at least 8 mg oral hydromorphone daily;
   - at least 25 mg oral oxymorphone daily; or
   - an equianalgesic dose of another opioid.

5. TIRF medicines are contraindicated in opioid-nontolerant patients.

6. TIRF medicines are contraindicated in the management of acute or postoperative pain, including headache/migraine and dental pain, or use in the emergency room.

7. Physicians should not convert patients on a µg per µg basis from another fentanyl medicine to a TIRF medicine, except for substitutions between a branded TIRF medicine and its generic equivalent.

8. Patients and their caregivers must be instructed that TIRF medicines contain a medicine in an amount that can be fatal in children, individuals for whom it is not prescribed, and those who are not opioid tolerant. All medicines must be kept out of the reach of children.

TIRF REMS Access program and accessibility to treatment

The TIRF REMS Access program is not meant to hinder the treatment of any patient who needs a ROO to manage their cancer breakthrough pain (cBTP). It is meant to help ensure that these drugs are used safely. If a patient falls outside of the TIRF REMS Access labeling guidelines, this author recommends that, if possible, a pain specialist familiar with this class of drugs be consulted if treatment with a ROO seems indicated.

The FDA does not expect that the TIRF REMS Access program will affect patient access to TIRF medicines. Having a single shared REMS for all of the TIRF medicines will make it easier for prescribers and pharmacies to participate in the TIRF REMS Access program, which is expected to improve patient access to, and safe usage of, ROOs [1].

References

1 FDA US Food and Drug Administration. Questions and answers: FDA approves a class Risk Evaluation and Mitigation Strategy (REMS) for transmucosal immediate-release fentanyl (TIRF) medicines. www.fda.gov/Drugs/DrugSafety/InformationbyDrugClass/ucm284717.htm. Updated January 5, 2012. Accessed February 1, 2013.
2 TIRF REMS ACCESS. TIRF REMS Access Program Home. What is the TIRF REMS Access Program? www.tirfremsaccess.com. Accessed February 1, 2013.
3 Anderson R, Saiers JH, Abram S, Schlicht C, et al. Accuracy in equianalgesic dosing. Conversion dilemmas. J Pain Symptom Manage. 2001;21:397-406.

Chapter 7

Summary

The rapid-onset opioids (ROOs) represent a major advance in the treatment of cancer pain. They are the first pain medications specifically targeted to treat cancer breakthrough pain (cBTP) and they are currently the only US Food and Drug Administration (FDA)-approved opioids that come close to matching the time course of rapidly onsetting cBTP. There are now a number of different ROOs available for the clinician to choose from, and informed use of this class of drugs can clearly enhance patient care. Every clinician who manages cancer-related pain should be facile at using these drugs.

D. R. Taylor., *Managing Cancer Breakthrough Pain*,
DOI: 10.1007/978-1-908517-83-8_7, © Springer Healthcare 2013

Appendix

Please see pages 96 and 97 for an overview on all currently approved rapid-onset opioids, at the time of this book's publication. More information on all of these rapid-onset opioids can be found in their respective package inserts and in this book, as specified in the following table's index column.

D. R. Taylor., *Managing Cancer Breakthrough Pain*,
DOI: 10.1007/978-1-908517-83-8, © Springer Healthcare 2013

Approved rapid-onset opioids

Drug	Formulation	Doses (µg)
ACTIQ® (US) (fentanyl citrate) oral transmucosal lozenge (OTFC)	transmucosal buccal lozenge on a stick	200, 400, 600, 800, 1200, 1600
FENTORA® (US) (fentanyl citrate) buccal tablet (FBT) Effentora® (EU) buccal tablet Fentanyl	buccal tablet with OraVescent® technology	100, 200, 400, 600, 800
ABSTRAL® (US) (fentanyl) sublingual tablet (FST)	sublingual tablet	100, 200, 300, 400, 600, 800
Lazanda® (US) (fentanyl) nasal spray PecFent® (EU) fentanyl pectin nasal spray (FPNS)	pectin-based nasal spray	100, 400
ONSOLIS® (US) fentanyl buccal soluble film (FBSF)	buccal film with BioErodible MucoAdhesive (BEMA™) delivery technology	200, 400, 600, 800, 1200
SUBSYS™ (US) fentanyl sublingual spray (FSS)	sublingual spray- 63.6% ethanol	100, 200, 400, 600, 800, 1200†, 1600†
INSTANYL® (EU) intranasal fentanyl spray (INFS)	nasal spray	50, 100, 200

Approved rapid-onset opioids. *Packaging varies to meet the needs of each patient's specific titration level; for more information on titration schemes, please see appropriate prescribing information per agent and the titration descriptions in the text (page numbers are listed in this table's index column); †Subsys is approved for use at 1200 µg and 1600 µg by combining lower doses (2 x 600 µg, 2 x 800 µg, respectively) to achieve these higher doses. Data from Actiq [package insert] [1], Abstral [package insert] [2], Fentora [package insert] [3], Effentora [package insert] [4], Instanyl [package insert] [5], Lazanda [package insert] [6], PecFent [package insert] [7], Onsolis [package insert] [8], Subsys [package insert] [9].

Packaging*	Generic form available	Index, page number
1 lozenge per blister package, 30 blister packages per shelf carton	Yes	OTFC, general information, 41 OTFC, titration, 43 OTFC, other opioids, 43
4 tablets per blister card, 7 blister cards per pack	Yes	FBT, general information, 44 FBT, titration, 47 FBT, comparative clinical trials, 47
100–400-µg doses in individually sealed blister packages, 12 or 32 tablets per package; 600- and 800-µg doses in individually sealed blister packages, 32 tablets per package	No	FST, general information, 48 FST, titration, 50 FST, other rapid-onset opioids, 50
8 100- or 400-µL sprays per 5.3-mL bottle, 1 or 4 bottles per carton	No	FPNS, general information, 50 FPNS, titration, 52 FPNS, other rapid-onset opioids, 53 FPNS, comparative clinical trials, 53
1 film per protective foil package, 30 foil packages per carton	No	FBSF, general information, 54 FBSF, titration, 56 FBSF, other rapid-onset opioids, 56
1 disposal bottle† per blister package, 6, 14, or 28 blister packages per carton	No	FSS, general information, 57 FSS, titration, 58 FSS, comparative clinical trials, 58
50-, 100-, and 200-µg doses in packs of 2, 6, 8, and 10 containers; also available in same strength multidose vials, 10 or 20 doses per vial	No	INFS, general information, 59 INFS, titration, 59 INFS, OTFC, 59

References

1   Actiq [package insert]. Frazer, PA: Cephalon, Inc; 2011.
2   Abstral [package insert]. Bridgewater, NJ: ProStrakan Inc.; 2012.
3   Fentora [package insert]. Frazer, PA: Cephalon, Inc.; 2011.
4   Effentora [package insert]. Maisons-Alfort, France: Cephalon France; 2012.
5   Instanyl [package insert]. Roskilde, Denmark: Nycomed Danmark ApS; 2012.
6   Lazanda [package insert]. Bedminster, NJ: Archimedes Pharma US Inc.; 2012.
7   PecFent [package insert]. Scandicci, Italy: Archimedes Development Ltd; 2012.
8   Onsolis [package insert]. Franklin Township, NJ: Meda Pharmaceuticals; 2012.
9   Subsys [package insert]. Phoenix, AZ: INSYS Therapeutics, Inc.; 2012.

Printed by Publishers' Graphics LLC
DBT131222.20.11.30